NOTES FROM A
BLACKBERRY

PALMETTO
PUBLISHING
Charleston, SC
www.PalmettoPublishing.com

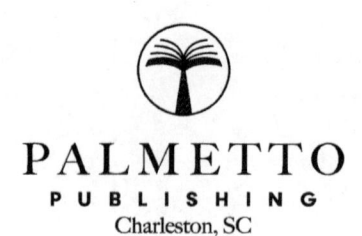

Copyright © 2024 by Julie Barth

All rights reserved

No portion of this book may be reproduced, stored in a retrieval system, or transmitted in any form by any means—electronic, mechanical, photocopy, recording, or other—except for brief quotations in printed reviews, without prior permission of the author.

Hardcover ISBN: 979-8-8229-4680-4
Paperback ISBN: 979-8-8229-3715-4

Notes From a
BLACKBERRY

Julie Barth

Preface

I wrote this story in the heat of the battle. So going back over it to reread, and in many ways relive, I thought long and hard about the things that I said: not just about me, but about others. When, back then, I finished writing the final page, and it said something about "happy endings", I really had hoped that the story and struggles would end there. But in life, the world keeps spinning. And in my life, sometimes things spin out of control and I am totally blindsided; other times I head into the wreckage, knowing full well what I am doing. Yet I always hope that I have, at the forefront of my mind, the best intentions of the people I love.

    I considered changing the narrative so as to be less "harsh" and "raw", and perhaps removing things that I said amidst the carnage, as I certainly did not want to hurt anyone's feelings. But illness makes you say, do, and perceive things in a way that isn't "normal". I have many times since Colin's death heard that I never grieved—but grieving is not a once-and-done thing.

    But that's the thing: when we talk with our "inside voice" we tell ourselves how we really feel and what OUR opinions are. Regardless if they are real, imagined, exaggerated, untrue, we speak from a dark place within our own minds—out from which we allow our emotions. Inside, we allow that voice to say what it wants, to yell if it wants, to be angry if it wants. But we control it on the outside, and perhaps some would say "thank God for that".

Illness has a way to bring out the worst in all of us. We are selfish, because although it might not be happening *to* us, it still is happening to us: because, like a pond with a rock touching the water, it's impact ripples out. And so it is okay to be selfish. Throughout this book, I tell my inner thoughts, my deepest regrets, my selfish decisions, my irrational thinking process, and yes, even the things that no one would ever want for someone else to hear.

I didn't change a word (well, the editor might have, because truth be told I am *horrible* with grammar), but the meaning of those words ring true. They are MY thoughts, not anyone else's, and I left them there on purpose.

Someone asked me the other day, "What is your objective in writing this story?" My answer was that, first, I wanted for the world to know of Colin's strength, courage, perseverance, and for everyone to know him the way that I did: the parts—amazing and genuine parts—that he showed to me and those around him. Secondly, I wrote it for Tayt. There was a reason that God put me in both of their ways, and it was to tell of their struggles, their true goodness, and the lessons that people are meant to learn from their short time together. What I realized just today—as I contemplated my writing of this book and putting it out into the universe to be scrutinized, judged, and perhaps (and almost assuredly for some) misunderstood—is that it is my responsibility to carry on with their courage.

If one person reads this and understands that illness isn't fair or rational, and sometimes God does not just give you what you can handle—He gives you far more—and as a result feels less horrible about their inside voice, and less ashamed of their anger and ugliness;

and if that one person therefore understands that it is human to react to impossible things with things you thought it impossible for yourself to do, then that is why God put me in their path, and on mine.

Try to be kinder to those in trauma, give people the benefit of the doubt, and please recognize that you cannot judge what goes on in someone's mind until you are privy to their inside voice: which you are not, yet God is.

God bless you Colin wherever you are, I will someday see you again . . .

Chapter One

Running—I'm always running. I run daily, incessantly, ever acquiring more mileage. Throwing on my shoes and hitting the pavement when I least feel like it, when I feel like my soul is going to break. Not an ounce of energy left to give to anyone, but I still run. I find within myself that last piece of adrenaline to get up and out the door every day. For if I didn't, if I stopped and I stood still, I would begin to feel things and see everything around me. I would see all that I am missing, all that is broken, all that is wrong. If I run, run to the point where I have nothing left, no feeling, no last piece of electricity in my body, then I am in a state of emptiness. Sometimes emptiness is the perfect feeling. When you are empty, there is nothing to regret, there is no guilt, there are no choices—there is just emptiness. That is how I feel: empty. I run with the intention of feeling that way. I run to get away from the things that I feel that will certainly take me away like a tidal wave. If I let things catch up with me, to overcome me, to make me anything less than empty, I will be swallowed whole. So I strap on those shoes, leave my world behind, and return when I feel nothing. That is what I want—to feel nothing.

Some say you can create reality. There are so many parts of me that are afraid that is true. I'm terrified that I really can create what is going on around me. I had known for so long that there would be some tragedy in my early years: except I always thought it was going to be me. I can remember when Jake, my oldest child, was a baby—and I felt no older than a baby myself: looking into the mirror with him, crying as I told him how sad I was that I would never watch him grow up. I always felt this impending doom, which now I feel on a continual basis. I don't know if it is from sheer guilt that I am not the one who's sick, or that my mind or my spirit knows that it is just a matter of time before I join Colin in the sickness that has overcome our lives, robbed me of my world, robbed us both of our very beliefs and souls. If it is true and we can create our own destiny, I am destined to create a life of misery. That is what I dream about. It's all I know.

I knew my father would die early. I knew that Colin, my young and full-of-life husband, would develop a terminal illness very early on. My "knowing" is filling me with self-doubt: with the possibility that I am not mentally well; with the possibility that making it up in my mind is making it real around me. I can't help but wonder (and worry about) why I know these things; why I feel something coming before it appears; why I can smell a situation, as if it is lingering in the air. It's not just a sense of global panic or anxiety, but one of truly knowing what's coming before the road has even begun to twist or turn—something like the mirrors that they put up around a bend in the road so that you can see what is coming at you in order to avoid it. The difference is, I am not able to avoid it. There is nothing to get me out of the line of fire or to stop it from coming directly at me.

Sometimes it feels like I'm creating it, like I'm inviting the drama. It sounds so egotistic, self-centered beyond imagination—I know, right? But it's more than déjà vu. It's so much more than that. When I see something unfold, I know from the start how it will end. So many times I have gone and seen movies—the ones that have the twists and turns, the ones that have you sitting on the edge of your seat—only to inevitably whisper to whomever I am with the exact ending: who did what, who killed who. I know from the outset what is going to happen, and am rarely wrong. The people around me get extremely annoyed with me, so I refrain from doing it now; but for years I wanted everyone to know that I actually did know the ending ahead of time. I needed for the person I was with to know that I had it all figured out, because otherwise anyone can leave the theater saying "I knew it was going to be that guy!", yet all the while their friends think to themselves *Yeah, sure you did.*

That's it. I know what will happen in my life before it starts. It is a curse, though I wouldn't go so far as to say I am psychic. Truth be told, I don't believe in them. Certainly, I believe that you can know things about people, places, and things around you that you are not supposed to know. I don't think that it is "psychic", though—I think it's just that you are open to and ready to receive information. There are signs everywhere, around ALL of us, not just a certain select few. Some people are just better able to tune in, to listen. I listen constantly, even when I don't want to hear. And it doesn't make it any easier when it comes true. There's no satisfaction in the "I told you so".

When I heard Katie Couric's husband died, I knew that day. *Literally* that day, I remember thinking, "That is going to be me. I am going to lose Colin". Almost like in the movie theater, where I had to prove I knew the end ahead of time, I wanted to tell someone about Colin so many years ago. But what would I gain by being right? There's no "winning" in being right on this one. Knowing what you shouldn't know is not a gift—it just brings on needless anxiety.

I am a truly analytical being. I look at a situation and I count the odds. If the odds are, or were ever, something that applied to my life, well, I would defy them. However, I wouldn't defy them in the "She beat the streets and became president" kind of way, but more in the "Are you kidding me? That *that many* bad things can happen in a row?" way. I feel like a sideshow freak, the "Unlucky Girl".

I don't know if I believe that there is one "God". If there is, he is a very busy being—and quite unfair, I might add—or there is a host of fates who have aligned this life for each of us to learn something. But what is the point of knowing ahead of time? I see the car accident, but there is nothing I can do to avoid it. Just knowing that it is going to happen has made me a distraught, and I guess hopeless, individual, as I see it continually unfolding at every turn.

Over the years many people have told me that I should write a book. I was hesitant because I sometimes feel like my life is just another life. I don't want people to judge me or my life; to judge my life as something to be pitied and talked about. But when Colin got sick, I realized that my life is like a car accident you don't want to see but are compelled to watch. It's as if I am standing in front of someone who is chomping away at their popcorn, waiting for the next twist or turn to make them laugh, cry, jump from their seat, invested in the outcome. I swear to you that no one could make our world up, nor would they want to! Everything that I write in this book happened.

I believe in the sheer odds of things. When I think about anything that could occur, I always turn to the law of odds. When I was pregnant for the first time, I thought for sure it had to be a boy. Everyone that I knew at the time was having a girl, so that meant I was going to have a boy. Because of the nature of odds, it had to even out; the world always has a yin and a yang, right?

If you see a train wreck, human nature provokes you to watch as much as you can before you look away. It's like playing chicken with your emotions. It gives you an odd sort of satisfaction at being in a front row seat, feeling part of it. Maybe it is the gladiator-spectator in all of us: enjoying the thrill of watching what the human spirit can endure, hoping for either outcome and not knowing which one will cause the bigger thrill, yet at the same time being ashamed and in denial that you are enjoying it all the same. That is what our life has been. It invokes fear, guilt, pleasure, and intrigue, and that is why I think our story should be told. It has an odd echo to it for all the wrong reasons, but it also shines through with the goodness of the human spirit.

When the hundredth person in my life said to me, "What more, Julie? What more could happen?" I pleaded with them to never ask that question again. I always felt like when you have the collective consciousness of so many people asking it, is almost like tempting the fates: daring them in some sadistic way; asking them to show us that they are capable of whatever they choose, even if it seems unimaginable.

Oddly, there is always a glimmer in their eyes that they're unaware of—excitement at the sheer prospect of there being more. I see what they won't admit to me or to themselves: that it is somewhat enjoyable, somewhat intriguing; that they feel some satisfaction in the fact they can watch from the passenger's seat and it isn't them. That they can watch on in horror and feel the comparison to where they are in life. We are giving them the very reason to feel better about their life, about themselves: a standard to gauge themselves against and then say, "At least we aren't the Barths", or "At least WE have our health". It's like they are mentally calculating their own odds, thinking *If it is happening to them, the odds of it happening to me are so much lower.* I know Colin also makes them vulnerable (the *It can happen to anyone, even me* feeling), but, when that feeling passes, they are left knowing it was not them, and they have gained a new perspective on how lucky they are, how lucky they are that they are not me. And so when you inevitably meet that person in your life who seems to deal with far more than their share of misery—the one that you would consider "unlucky" or unable to catch a break—don't ask the fates out loud what more could happen. Look around you and you can see their power.

My eleven-year-old asked me yesterday: if there was a cup in front of me that was half-filled with liquid, what would I call it? I know it's supposed to be some sort of psychological determination of how I perceive the world, be it positive or negative, but I don't subscribe to that notion. I told him that it all depends on what state it begins in. If I started with a full glass, then I would see it as half empty; if I started with an empty glass, I would see it half full. That is my perspective on our lives. I know that in developing countries where disease is commonplace, one would consider thirty-five to be a ripe old age. It's like how, when someone dies in their nineties, we see it as justifiable, not a tragedy; we say they lived a full life. So, to someone who doesn't have food to eat, our glass is definitely half full. We were born into privilege. We were born with a full glass—a life expectancy of seventy-two and a half years, children free from diseases like polio, pleurisy, you name it—and then someone emptied our glass. I am still thankful to have half a glass, but I can't help wishing it was full, you know? Of course my child shook his head, as if asking, "Can't you just answer the question like other parents do?" That's his perspective: *Can't we just be like other families?* I wish that I could tell him, "Yes, honey, eventually we will be like other families; eventually our lives will maintain some semblance of normalcy and we won't be living in this weird alternate universe where we're looking for the cameras".

In some respects I completely understood and was somewhat frightened by the Jim Carrey movie *The Truman Show*. That is how I feel sometimes: that at some point someone is going to jump out and say, "We've been completely screwing with you! Of course this isn't your REAL life; no one's life can endure THAT MUCH crazy shit . . . We were just taping it for entertainment purposes!". Unfortunately, our situation in life is not funny, and I don't know that it will ever be. In his eleven years Jake has lived so much, endured so much, I sometimes wonder how these situations will impact him growing up.

The first real memory that I have of thinking this—not just the flashes or the smells, but the whole situation—is that I remember Jake turning eight and me thinking, "Okay, now it counts. Now he will remember everything that he endures, everything he encounters". I remember thinking how I'd better pick myself up and fly right, because from that point on it was being recorded; that this would come back to life in twenty years should my children be reminiscing over the years of torture and insults they endured from their childhood and from me. *From this point on*, I thought, *I better watch myself.* I found myself bending over backwards, taking Jake to every Sesame Street live show, or Blue's Clues (you name it, we went to it). Yet the things he still remembers most are when I was ten minutes late picking him up, or when I forgot his gym uniform. The negatives seem to burn into the soul so much more rapidly and vividly than the positive things we encounter.

I have hesitated to write what follows down because I don't know where to begin. It would be like stopping to describe an avalanche. Do you describe it at the top of the mountain where it truly began, or midway down where it starts to impact the things around it? I am going to start at the very top and then skip to the highlights.

*

When I myself was eight, I remember moving to a new home in a new town. Mind you, it was only twenty minutes from my old house, but to an eight-year-old it might as well have been Egypt. Now, looking back, that seems so insignificant, because you really only remember bits and pieces anyway. You remember scents and sounds, but not really locations—just the people involved. It's like reading the CliffsNotes version instead of the novel. Nor do I remember much about the first year at my new school—though I do remember the day I first laid eyes on Colin Barth.

It was the late 70s and his mother definitely believed in the fashion of the times. He had a long shag haircut like Dudley Moore; more of a wave across his forehead. When he would sweat, it would cause the flip in the front of his hair to drape just over the kind of eyes that you could see the world reflecting in. He had a distinctive mole on his nose: perfectly placed, as if he'd been kissed by an angel; a bronze color to his flawless skin; and his teeth were beautifully perfect, yet way too big for his growing mouth. Still, the thing that would stop you dead in your tracks were those soulful and bottomless blue eyes.

Hardened by time and by the complexity that life brings to us as adults, it is almost impossible to remember that feeling of instant love. The feeling whereby you think you are most assuredly going to throw up right there and then, yet then waves of euphoria hit: like an electrical surge of the most beautiful excitement that you can imagine—excitement that you feel in your toes first, next your stomach, and then finally you feel your heart racing, as if it is going to jump right out of your chest. Unfortunately, that feeling of complete and utter elation is wasted on youth. As with most things, you don't realize how truly miraculous it is until you don't remember what it feels like. Then you spend the rest of your time here on earth chasing it, complaining about not having it, wishing you could have it for just one more minute. It's like the drug of a lifetime and you don't know that you won't have it again, so you don't know to appreciate it when it happens. That is the very love that I felt for Colin, running around that schoolyard during those spring days after I moved to my new surroundings.

Those feelings; the hopefulness; the possibilities of having my feelings returned, were always followed up by the note that would be inevitably passed when we were supposed to be doing our schoolwork. The previous night would be spent trying to write the perfect note: the one that would be answered just the way I wanted it to be. If I made that note into some sort of subliminal, perfect mind-controller, it would come back with the answers that I longed for. I would devise notes so incredibly simple that they would always be answered, yet those answers could then be read into whichever way I wanted. Most of the time it was either a statement with a "true" or a "false" to be circled, or one carefully worded to be finished in a way that would make tears of joy come to my eyes. Those were the kind of notes of manipulation that we all pored over. No texts, no instant gratification; just a note, passed with the hopes it would be answered—and answered in a way that would make our heart soar, not in a way that would make our whole world fall apart.

I was always mesmerized by the intensity in Colin's eyes. They were like looking at the sun: something that you want desperately to be able to look at directly—to look into, to figure out what it truly holds, how it truly looks, what secrets it hides—yet the intensity is too much and you end up having to look away. To this day, when you look into Colin's eyes you feel as if you can peer right into his soul. And his heart is so open you probably are. Those are the eyes I saw that day when I met him. He had the eyes of an eighty-year-old spirit: the way you can look into an older person's eyes and you are so aware of what they are thinking and where they have been. He seemed to have so much going on for an eight-year-old. His soul seemed to be so far much older than his body. That is how I remember my husband when I met him twenty-eight years ago. He was quiet; in fact that's what I remember most, his quietness. He wasn't a typical boy: rambunctious, loud, trying to get attention by being the most boisterous or the most boastful. He got attention through his withdrawal. Only years later did I begin to see the motivations behind our younger lives. Only years later did I hear the stories of the things that he was introduced to way too young in life. Only years later was I able to piece together the loneliness of an eight-year-old who was ridiculed and dismissed by his twin brothers. To this anyone would probably comment, "Well, who wasn't dismissed by their brothers and sisters? Who wasn't lonely?" My memory holds lots of people who were not; or perhaps lots of people who were, yet who had the ability to block it out. But Colin was guided so severely by his sensitivity, his kindness, his awareness of those around him. It was as if he could feel the ridicule of others. He walked not only a day in someone else's shoes, but a lifetime, constantly walking in the hearts of others. He seemed so pained by what he saw and what he felt. He felt for others what they did not feel themselves.

That is where we met: on a playground full of bell-bottoms, four square and shuttle races, its monkey bars shaped like domes. It seems like a lifetime ago, but in a weird way also like just a couple of pages' turning.

Colin was always kind of a sad soul. He was a loner; well-liked enough and with many surface friends, yet he always stood out. Not because he was awkward or unkempt or picked his nose—but because he knew too much about life. He knew so much about the complexities of the things around him. He was popular and handsome, and would never lack for girls wanting to be with him, but there was something in him that was special: something so guarded and hidden away behind those steel-blue eyes. To this day you can feel his extraordinary presence from merely being in the same room. You hang on his every word. You are both excited (and, yes, sometimes extremely insulted) by what he has to say, but in the end you know it's real, you know it's honest. There are not words wasted or time to kill when you are with Colin. You are given his unfiltered honesty, whatever it is.

In those early years Colin spent much of his time in search of attention. And there were times he would do some pretty stupid things. I suppose it was a cry for help: something we all may have done, but just on a grander scale. Immediately after Colin was diagnosed with pancreatic cancer, I was having dinner with a couple of girls from grade school, friends of both Colin's and mine. In fact, it is hard to tell who met who first because we all are so intertwined. The drinks started flowing and I started telling the story of a young, eleven-year-old Colin in a fight with our girlfriend Stacey. Not just any fight, but one of those kicking and slapping fights. Stacey was the victor and to the ground Colin fell. He lay on that school playground for so long that the bell eventually started summoning everyone else in. And he was yelling "My pancreas! My pancreas!" as he grabbed his stomach. It sent a chill through all three friends, that we all remembered this. We all recalled his words, and we all thought about it instantaneously the day we found out about the cancer; somehow it now felt like a foreboding. Who at the age of eleven even knows what a pancreas is? I know it is probably just a coincidence, but it's an eerie, unnerving, unsettling coincidence at that.

Those were different days. There were no anti-bullying campaigns, and no lessons on self-esteem. If you competed in a sport, someone won and someone lost: that was the cruel reality of our lives.

We didn't have baby-proofing, or child-resistant medicine bottles. We didn't have screws on our battery covers, or covers for our electrical outlets. But somehow we survived. We learned from our mistakes, and that which did not literally kill us, made us stronger.

We have lived our lives believing exactly that—that which didn't kill us would make us stronger. But that's not the case with cancer. That which does not kill us can rob our souls and our hopes. That which does not kill us weakens us to the brink and changes our lives. Yes, it is true that it strengthens our appreciation, our relationships, perhaps even our understanding of the true meaning of life—but it does nothing but insult to our physical being. It takes a toll on our emotions and our physicality that can never be repaired. I guess it's in the eye of the beholder, but this experience seems so unnecessary and has taught me nothing more than I have already learned. This experience will not make me stronger, just more gun-shy, more scared of losing, more fragile, and more vulnerable . . . not strong.

We would soon finish our years at North Barrington Elementary and move to middle school, and in doing so part ways for what seems like lifetimes. Though before we did, I love to look back on and tell the story about how Colin was my first kiss—though the story only gets as good a reaction when I add that I was not his! (After all, he had twin brothers five years older and was on a much faster track than I.)

We went to the sixth-grade fun fair together. It was by far the biggest day in any North Barrington student's world. As sixth graders, we were all giddy with the prospect of going with a member of the opposite sex. It would be my first date—and with my inability to make good decisions, I accepted two offers. Evidently to my twelve-year-old mind I was being kind: spreading myself around, not having to let anyone down by saying no. *I don't want to make anyone unhappy*, I thought, *there's enough of me to go around.* Only years later did I realize that I impacted Colin at all.

The truth is that I have always, and continue to this day, struggled to tell anyone no. I am so fearful of the repercussions of the word "no" that I really have a hard time saying it. Yes, many times it has come back to bite me in the ass; and you would think that, after thirty-seven years of it backfiring at least seventy percent of the time, I would just learn to say no. But that is one of my major flaws (one of many, I suppose): that inability to ever appear the bad guy. I have lied, cheated, and hustled my way into never having to say no. I offer up things that I don't really want to, I make plans I don't intend to keep. I guess I am a product of my upbringing. There was so much strife in my family; we went through periods of time where my parents did nothing but argue. It was like a fight in a back alley: the struggle is almost unbearable to hear, but what is more unnerving is the silence when the scuffle is over.

In the midst of those "back alley" fights, I became the peacemaker—believing, quite self-centeredly, that I had the power to change it. I believed that if I just made everything nice and easy for everyone, my parents would find their way back to each other. I never wanted to see them unhappy or disappointed. Those are the feelings that I carried with me and would continue into my own relationships.

So, because I was too selfish to say no to anyone at the time, I went to the first half of the fun fair with Colin and the second half with another boy. It seemed like the perfect solution. I remember so clearly when I kissed Colin goodbye. I can still feel the kiss on my lips, and I wished I could have spent a lifetime more with him. I remember not wanting to leave him; not wanting to move on to Jeff, the second boy. I wish I could've frozen that moment, relived it over and over again—not just in my mind, but really tasted his lips, smelled his sweet breath. I even remember the look on his face as he turned to leave. He looked at me as if pleading, "Don't go, don't walk away right now, we have so much more to do together". That is the look that I remembered—perhaps the same look that I give when I visit him in the hospital. My soul pleading with him to fight this, win over this cancer, stay with me.

But I remember that look. Oddly enough I hadn't until just now, imagining that moment in time. I had forgotten the look he gave me as he left me standing at the front of the school, and I wish I could go back there and never let him walk away. We had so much time that we should have spent together. Little did I know that back then. Yet, in a strange sort of way, I did know.

I remember, at twelve years old, talking with one of my best friends about marrying Colin one day, and practicing writing "Julie Barth" over and over. I knew somewhere in my heart that this was just the beginning of my life as Julie Barth. I can remember it like it was yesterday: writing a whole page of my eventual name, knowing that it felt more right than writing my own name at the time. I remember writing it, looking down at it and feeling an odd sensation that it was a way of knowing what life had in store. It was my soul telling me that I was going to be a part of Colin Barth for my whole life; he would always be tied to me; he would always define me: what my life was before he was in it, while he was in it, and long, long after he had exited it. Looking back, I knew it was just the beginning—I just had no idea of what that entailed.

The fun fair was our final goodbye to elementary school. In middle school, Colin immediately knew just about everyone from years of different sports. All the boys knew each other and he settled in fairly easily. In fact, when I think of middle school, I don't remember really seeing him at all. For two years we attended the same school and probably passed each other daily, but almost pretended not to know one another.

Middle school was not so easy for me. I had a hard time: my insecurities, there from the start, really hit an all-time high.

During those years, my parents started growing further apart. My mother began her own career as a local real estate agent and was very good at it. I think that my dad—who never had the courage to try anything more than janitorial professions, even with a college degree—disliked her success. Within a couple of years of working in real estate my mother was in the million-dollar club, earning more than him and enjoying her life outside of him.

Meanwhile, while she found a job that she really enjoyed, he found a secretary that he really enjoyed.

Looking back on my parents' relationship, I think they were always fond of one another, but I don't think that they really enjoyed each other. Whereas, since Colin and I married, I don't think there is a soul in the world that I would rather go out with, day or night. I remember when my friends would have ladies' nights, or go on vacation with "the girls". I just wanted to be with Colin. I loved the time we shared together. The times that we went out, the times we spent laughing and talking until the wee hours of the morning: those are the nights that I will remember forever.

So what was once teenage angst and anger at both parents—or maybe more toward my father—over the years has turned to pity. Pity that I don't think either of them ever found someone that they truly enjoyed being around. They were like an old pair of shoes, but ones that you put on only because newer alternatives are too costly. They stayed together as long as they did because it was too expensive not to.

Thus my middle school years were marred with poor (if any) attendance, avoidance behavior, insecurity, fear, and angst—*a lot* of angst. Colin and I had both moved on to bigger crowds than those in our tiny grade school. He started excelling in sports and, well, I started my years of trying to be inconspicuous, really trying to disappear.

I was an awkward teenager. I always believed myself to be about one hundred pounds more than I was, and I felt awkward and self-conscious. I remember wearing my jacket around school, day after day: never taking it off because of my fear of being too fat, or not having the right clothes. Every day was torture trying to fit in. Every day was an attempt to just get through the day unscathed, with no one mad at me or talking behind my back. Truth be told, people probably couldn't be bothered with me—in fact, they probably didn't even know I existed—and I was okay with that. But the thought of someone not liking me? Well, that was too much. Someone not saying "Hi" to me in the halls would lead to days filled with wondering what I had done. I lived many years—and probably still do—trying desperately to get everyone to like me. I find that I judge my worth through the eyes of others. I depend so much on what other people think of me in order to decide how I think of myself, and that insecurity, in an atmosphere like middle school, makes a breeding ground for misery.

However, either now or looking back, you would never know that from the outside. I have an aura of self-assuredness that radiates outward—it's just someone forgot to tell my soul.

*

I can't tell you how many people over the years have marveled at how "strong" I am. Strength is such a funny term. If by "strong" they mean I can smile and pretend that I am fine, then I'm the strongest human alive. If by "strong" you mean that I live each day in terror of what goes on around me and try just to get through the day making everyone around me happy, then yes, I am strong. But if you define "strong" as truly believing not only in yourself but also what you mean to others, then I am anything but strong.

I remember, shortly after Colin was diagnosed with cancer, many times when people were saying I was a rock, to which I replied: "No, I am more like an egg. I seem strong when you touch my outside, but am a mess on the inside. Don't break or crack that outer shell or you will be mopping up pieces of my soul off the ground." It has taken me all my thirty-seven years to realize how I come across to others. There is a huge discrepancy between who I am and who I seem to be. Reflecting back, it took me many years to build up this façade—only to wish that I hadn't. That's what we all are: bundles of years of insult and rewards. We all begin with a soul, which is then turned and reshaped and turned again, until one day we wake up and realize that we are not what we used to be.

It's like keeping a bottle of wine in a carefully guarded place, only to open it up on a special occasion and realize it has turned into vinegar. I don't think that my soul is vinegar, but it's definitely not the originally packaged fine wine I was born as. My experiences, and what I have had to do, and the decisions I have made because I felt like I had no choice—they have left parts of me hollow, soured, undrinkable. They were decisions that I had to make, and I still believe that. They were actions that I had to take; insignificant things that I had to care about, no doubt—but that doesn't stop them from changing not only who you are, but who you think you are, and the way you feel about yourself. It's like when people without children say, "my child will never . . ." I have sworn that I would never do things, and then had to completely settle up with fate to take those words back. I have had to look at situations that originally looked black and white and add gray to them. That is what life has made me do. I am not proud of all my decisions, but if I ever start to second-guess them . . . again, you would be picking up pieces of me off the floor.

Life changes us and alters us into being people and doing things that we don't want to or never imagined we would. Sometimes I lie in bed asking for forgiveness from so many people, souls, God—praying that I was not just being selfish in saying I had no choice, but that I really made the right choice.

Chapter Two

When you sit in this room filled with cancer patients, bald heads, nagging wives, and you just stop to listen, you get an eerie sense of IV machines pulsating to the same beat. They're almost like an army of misled officers, trudging wearily into battle. Imagine these troops knew that their efforts were fruitless. Imagine someone saying to them, "Okay, men, get your ineffective swords together and let's just try to keep them from winning for as long as we can. They know that eventually they will take you, with no real meaning for the battle to begin with, but try your best."

That is the morale of this place. That is the battle cry of these awful ineffective machines as they inject their ineffective poison into the veins of hundreds of people. Prior to Colin's diagnosis, I was not privy to the actual logistics of having cancer; those that any survivor or otherwise would attest to. The whole thing is so very methodical, yet surreal. They make you line up like sheep. They call your name, almost like it's a number. You take a seat in a room that at first glance looks like an emergency room, except the booths are just tiny enough to fit you, an IV, and (if you are lucky enough), someone who gets you food while you are hooked up. This is no emergency room, though. This is an unreal room, where you have a seat, take your poison, and then are directed to leave promptly so the next person can continue and do the same. Everyone there seems mindless. The first time I went, I remember feeling sick to my stomach. It is a room full of despair and hope, baldness and nausea, suffering. You can literally smell the suffering; you can taste it, you can feel it, you can hear it. It looks like a refugee camp, like a developing country in the middle of a hospital. It is unbelievable. I can try to describe it, but it's almost like what was said of Ground Zero: you can't even imagine the devastation until you are standing and looking over it. That's the chemo ward. That is what you see on what I call "chemoday".

*

By the time we got to high school, Colin was dating one of my friends. I would see him in the hallways, and I remember every time I saw him I would get that giddy feeling in the pit of my stomach. But at that point I felt he was way out of my league. And truth be told he was.

I remember him so vividly: the locker I would see him standing next to, coming out of English class—I even remember that it was seventh period. It's funny how the mind can hold onto such apparently trivial events. I guess they seemed trivial, up until I realized that those moments are the very moments that I have frozen in my brain. They're the moments of Colin that I will never lose: his liveliness, his youth, the way he used to make me feel, the happiness that I felt just when he was near me.

The high school years were not so good to me either. As I say, my parents were not soulmates; they were two people who decided to get married and made a life of it. My mom wanted to travel and my father was a homebody. He wanted nothing more than to stay home and watch television, he had no sense of adventure. Any sense of it that his soul had ascertained was quickly squashed by his many fears. Fear was the one common denominator with which my father guided everything in his life. He was afraid to die, though even more afraid to actually live. If he did live, and enjoyed it, then when it was time to die he would miss it far too much. I watched him there, on the sidelines of life: wanting to join in, wanting to live, yet held back by a force that he wore like a fort. It was always evident to me, as well as to anyone who knew my mother, listened to my mother, or talked to my mother, that somewhere along the way she had pitied my father enough to marry him—enough, in her mind, to conjure up her sympathies and squash her wanderlust to allow him that one pleasure: the pleasure of marrying her.

In the midst of all this, I struggled ferociously to gain attention—any attention. I fought against invisibility by being overly sensitive to everyone's needs. I thought that, if I could just please everyone, then they would love me, they would notice me, they would care about me. My parents both wore their misery like a badge of courage. To me, it was a badge of cowardice: fear of ever wanting or trying for anything that wasn't easy or comfortable; fear of giving of your self; of being alive in the moment—being alive at all.

Knowing that Colin already had a girlfriend, and feeling as if I had missed my chance, I did what any immature young woman would do: I ignored him, forgot about him, and disliked him. Why? Well, really for no reason other than my own pride—but is there ever any other reason at that coming-of-age period? It wasn't until years later when I realized that there was never a single moment in time that I could remember Colin being anything but gracious and kind (yes, brutally honest, which can be hurtful, but never on purpose). Life lends to the ill an erasure of one's prior faults and indiscretions. It allows us to again overwrite someone's past, and the history of who they were prior to illness. But I am not doing that here. Colin truly is such a kind soul. A gentle, sensitive, and caring soul. I am sorry I missed all those years when I rewrote him to make my own insecurities vanish.

We met up again years later when I was living in the city. I graduated with a degree in psychology, but as anyone with a psych degree knows, the starting salary in that industry will not pay your bills, so I took a position as an executive assistant/graphic designer downtown Chicago. Colin had graduated college a year after me and he happened upon a bar in Chicago where every night in your twenties turns into a high school reunion if you are from a radius of one hundred miles. He walked into the bar, walked over by me, and I could hear his newly acquired Mississippi accent. I remember being so cruel: commenting how he was the same old Colin and that he would never change, as he handed his chair over to my friends. I ridiculed his accent as fake and stupid; I picked on his hairstyle; talked of stories I had heard about him, the drugs I heard he did—you name it, I was bringing it to light. He merely looked at me and smiled the most heartwarming smile, as if he was actually happy to see me. Here was this guy who I had rewritten in my mind to have done so much harm to me. (How, to me specifically, I am not sure; but the insult to my ego from him not acknowledging me had made me bitter.) Yet he had no bitterness. He was in fact very happy to see me, to talk to me, to catch up with me. I thought he had long since forgotten me, the pimply-faced girl who wanted so badly to have his attention in high school the way I had in elementary school. But he had no idea, and his memories of me were done away with—he was just glad to say hi and reconnect. Not until years after we got together did I know that I even affected him in elementary school. His brothers had seen me walk away with another date, and had made a spectacle of it after I had done so. He had every right to begrudge me, yet he never did.

I remember nothing more of the evening other than, by night's end, letting a little bit of my guard down; ever so slowly, ever so carefully. And how, from that point onward, we became inseparable: like two childhood friends being reacquainted. It was as if I had been missing my right arm all those years we were apart and I didn't even realize it. When you get good at doing things on your own you forget how nice and essential it is to have an extra appendage. That's what Colin is to me: he is an appendage. Of course, most of the time you can survive without it; but it's always different, and you have the phantom of it, which reminds you of what you are missing. Colin was that thing in my life I had been missing.

I had been dating another guy for over three years, just about the nicest guy anyone could know. We had talked seriously about getting married, but something just didn't feel right. I remember how, months after Colin and I met back up, Colin would just come to my apartment to hang out. Or we would go out together for drinks. Truth be told, that first month we went out every night. At the time things with Sean were dying down and we were almost beating a dead horse, yet I still hadn't been ready to end it.

Colin and I used to stay up all night laughing and drinking and talking. I don't think I have ever talked to someone the way that we did, even long before we were officially dating. We really were just friends at the time.

Although Colin worked downtown, he still lived in the suburbs, so he would come over after work and he would stay over, though nothing ever happened between the two of us. I remember one night in particular when he came downtown to go to dinner. We had had a couple—probably too many—to drink, and we decided to go up on top of the roof deck of my apartment. At the time we lived right in the heart of Lincoln Park; "we" being me, my friend from elementary school (Colin's friend as well), and another girl from Kansas. Our apartment faced the lake and we were right across the street from a famous children's hospital. I remember, that night, just sitting up there and having a real heart-to-heart. We were talking about what we wanted to do with our lives, where we saw our lives heading. I remember distinctively Colin saying that he wanted to travel.

He said he never wanted to stay put or be grounded—and I remember thinking that, even if I ever did see us dating or getting together, then our remaining together would not be on the cards. If there is one thing I am not, it is a traveler. I am a homebody. I wanted nothing more than to settle down, find a home, and never leave it. It was at that moment that I thought a lifetime together would never happen for us. But after all these years, I realize that he gave it up for me. He gave up the travel, the never staying put. He stayed put. Because that is what I wanted.

I think it was that night—the first night, when we kissed, the kiss of a lifetime, up on a rooftop deck with no guards, no borders, dangerous as it was beautiful—that our lives together began. We quickly moved in together (well, he moved in with me), and that is probably where the avalanche began.

I was working as a graphic designer, or maybe it was an executive assistant. For any woman who started a career in the nineties, "executive assistant" was really another term for secretary—only it required a college degree and it had a false promise of promotion behind it. When all was said and done, it went nowhere but to being a higher executive assistant (secretary). Colin was clerking at the Board of Trade. His sisters had started out there, and Colin was following in their footsteps. He was working for a firm that was allowing him to learn the ropes. He worked about three hours a day. Granted, he made only about $5 an hour; but he loved—and when I say loved, I mean *loved*—every minute of it.

After about a year of clerking—wherein he made many mistakes, and each day that he was welcomed back was a blessing—he started trading on the floor, all by himself. Many times in our lives, we have had roles that we were not prepared for. It's like how years after you have your children, you realize one day that not only did you have NO idea what you were doing, but all those years that you thought your mom did, she didn't either. It's an odd feeling when you think about your own age, and think that your mother was probably younger than you are at that moment, and you thought she knew everything. Maybe she had taken some sort of lessons. Nope, she was winging it too—and still is.

That was Colin's trading. He picked me up from work one day early on in our relationship, beaming. I still remember the smile, from ear to ear, as he handed me his trading notes. I was working in Libertyville, an outlying suburb far from our home in Chicago, and commuting three hours a day in a beat-up old Honda Prelude. He had had his first truly successful day.

When he was clerking, he would frequently come home from a long day, upset that one of the traders had yelled at him over "something stupid", some inconsequential mistake that he had made. So they lost thousands? It wasn't his fault, he would insist. Unfortunately, what goes around comes around, and I would have to remind him of those conversations after he became a trader—remind him how he had thought it was inconsequential when it wasn't his money, just a "little mistake". Yet in those early days I began to think that he didn't have a clue what he was doing. One day he would come home on cloud nine; the next, he would be devastated. It was a career of professional gambling, but he loved it.

After about six months of his trading and us not being able to pay the rent despite me working overtime, I sat him down and said to him: "I think it's time to take a different job. I don't think you know what you are doing, and even if you do, how many people actually become millionaires at the Board of Trade?" All I had known of there was either people who made a mediocre living, or those friends whom had quickly come and gone: young traders who played fast and loose—one minute they were worth millions, the next blown-out and looking for a new profession. Colin, to his credit, was hanging in, but I didn't know how much of the ups and downs he could take. I was afraid that the accumulation of being in that stressful state—day after day, year after year—would take its toll on him. But he insisted he loved it, and I never brought up quitting the profession again.

Over the years he would have periods where he would say he needed to get out because he couldn't take it anymore, but he always felt like he wasn't qualified to do anything else. He would try for maybe a month: he would get his resume together, buy a new suit (at least one a year, and which would never be worn), talk to people about positions within their company; and then, after the angst was over—after the realization that he could do what he was doing—the suit would be shelved and he would go back down to the Board of Trade.

*

He has never realized how intelligent he is and how good he is with people. He sees himself in such a limited light. His real dream was to be a teacher; but, as with many of the decisions in his life, he didn't think teaching would earn a good enough living for us. He wanted to have a couple of good years, make a whole lot of money, and then he could pursue his dreams. As any young person does, he believed that he had endless time. There was always time in the future to do what he wanted, so in the present he did what he thought was good for everyone else. Even after he got sick, he turned to me one day and said, "When this is all over, I am going back to school and I'm going to become a teacher". The dream never left him—he left it.

*

Those first years we lived together were some really fun times: filled with so many new things, out on our own, finding our way together. Our apartment was cool by Chicago standards. It was well off the beaten path, in what felt like the "older" area (not that the buildings were old, but the inhabitants were). We had moved from the crazy life of recent college graduates to being an up-and-coming couple. The apartment was unique; I still remember it to this day. It was quite large, with two bedrooms (well, one was really a loft that we used as a bedroom), with a lower area and a dining room and kitchen.

There was only one drawback—well, okay, maybe a thousand small drawbacks—in that it was a pit. The landlord apparently had inherited it from someone, and was bound and determined to milk it until it collapsed. It had critters living in the ceiling, duct tape on the carpeting, and I was sure it had asbestos throughout—you know, that kind of place. That was our first apartment. Nevertheless, WE LOVED EVERY MINUTE OF IT!

Colin called me at work one day while getting ready to head to work himself. He told me that he was wearing a towel and heard a scurrying sound in the ceiling above him. As he looked up, pieces of ceiling started to fall onto his face and into his eyes. As he squinted and rubbed his eyes, trying desperately to see what was going on, he saw a squirrel's claw appear. He said he saw one claw break through slightly, then another one, and then it backed away. He stared even harder, and tried to get closer, at which point the squirrel poked its head directly into the hole made by its claws. I always pictured that situation like it was computer-animated: Colin, looking up; and the squirrel, talking down to him.

We called John the landlord to tell him about the inhabitants in the ceiling. He was too cheap to actually do the right thing and thought it was silly to involve animal control. So he and one of his buddies went into the attic and covered up the holes so that the animals couldn't go in or out. Colin and I lived in that apartment for an entire summer with the smell of corpses baking in the attic. It must have smelled like a serial killer's home, yet no one called. Eventually, I suppose we just stopped smelling it.

One day Colin decided to have his parents over for dinner. When Colin and I first started hanging out together, we would go to his parents' house for Sunday dinners. They lived on a beautiful estate with a pool, and after a long weekend of drinking and partying and eating junk it was so nice to spend the day poolside and then have his mother cook us dinner. When I say that the dinners Diana made were incredible, that just doesn't even come close to describing them. They were straight out of the Martha Stewart magazine. In fact, I think my mother-in-law could teach her a couple of "good things". To Diana, Colin's mother, every meal was an event. Every meal had "the essentials", which at my home would have been interpreted as a glass of milk. At the Thomas', it meant multiple courses, a ton of fresh herbs, and always perfection.

Diana was a woman who made every occasion a real occasion. There was no such thing as "pizza night", or getting together for a casual dinner. Everything was always adorned, fussed over, and over-the-top, though never in an obnoxious way. Somehow all of her planning and hard work looked natural and seamless. Diana had been diagnosed in her early forties with ovarian cancer. She'd had persistent stomach issues, which continued to fall on deaf ears with her physician, until it got so bad that at a certain point they ended up bringing her in for "exploratory surgery". Four hours later, the family was told that she had stage four cancer that had metastasized pretty much everywhere. When they opened her up, it was described to me as if they had set free a brush fire. At the time she was given only a ten percent chance of making it post-surgery, and was never supposed to survive more than six months. Every day, every event, every breath to her was one that she didn't take for granted; she celebrated the big and small occasions as a victory for even being there.

Being at that house made me feel like I was something "less"—a fake at the country club wearing a borrowed dress, to whom someone had tried to explain the complexities of country club living, but who never really had the class or the upbringing to pull it off. So many times, I felt like I was uncultured. I wasn't sure what fork to use; didn't know what cilantro, or basil, or, well, what any herb was, nor what you were supposed to do with them. I was constantly trying to play the part, so afraid that I would be found out as a girl who grew up relatively poor with a janitor for a father and a home that was the size of their pool house.

To this day whenever people remark about my decorating or my cooking, I feel ashamed and like I am somehow cheating someone when they use words like "eloquent" or "beautiful" or "gifted". Those words make me think *If they really knew me, really knew how I put it together, what I used to cook it, they wouldn't think so,* or otherwise *They are just being nice. They must not know who I really am, what I am really made of inside.*

When I found out Colin had invited his parents to our apartment for dinner, I was horrified. No matter what I did to that apartment, it was fun, spacious, but *not* elegant or beautiful. I was embarrassed to have them come to our little place. I wanted to make sure that the apartment was perfect. I took the day off of work and started cleaning it from top to bottom—but, just as if I was putting steak sauce on Spam, there was no way of making our little abode anything more than what it was: a glorified bachelor and bachelorette pad.

When I took the day off work, I woke up wondering what I was best at cooking. I tried to decide what I could feed his parents that would even come close to their dinners. Of course there was nothing, so I thought I would go "eclectic". Can't go wrong with eclectic, right? First thing that morning I went to work making some chop suey-like concoction. I believe it required a phone call to my mother; and, looking back on it, that was just plain silly. When I was growing up, my mom's soups and stews always involved biting down on something hard and unrecognizable. Why I decided to consult her . . . well, I suppose it was just the proverbial "mom call".

All day long my concoction of whatever I decided to add (to this day, I have no idea) stewed. As dinner approached, I went to stir the "stew"—only to return to the living room to find Colin sitting with his parents and on the telephone ordering pizza.

After reexamining the entire situation, I know now that Colin was trying to protect me. He knew that whatever was brewing in that pot—whatever meat and extras I had conjured up—would likely just lead me to being embarrassed and considering the entire day a disaster. He was trying to save me from my own mess; to clean it up, make it right. That's who Colin was. He always let me tell my stories from my side without interjecting with his own. He knew I needed to validate the mess that I had made and tried to clean up. He knew

I needed to feel like my efforts were not a waste. He also knew the fallout of my own insecurities when things didn't go the way that I thought they would. He had the forethought to see the letdown that would ensue the day after the "chop suey" had been consumed. He probably knew that I would be judging his parents' every reaction, and analyzing and stressing out about it. He loved me enough to take the blame for being insensitive if that was the way it came across. He always had my back. He always thought about me, about the aftermath of the decisions I made—even when I did not.

It was late summer, a couple of months after we finally settled into living together, and I was sitting on the couch watching television.

About a month earlier, Colin had come home after spending the night out with his brother, to announce that we had given living together our best shot, but it just wasn't working. What was most curious about this was that nothing had happened. He had left the apartment the night before in positive spirits, said "Love you" as he headed out the door—yet here he now was: standing in front of me, assuring me that he would give me a couple of weeks to find another place.

Even as I subsequently said goodbye to Colin, vacating the apartment once those weeks had passed, I suppose I never really believed that it was over. I assumed that somewhere in his heart he would realize his mistake, and he would call and tell me that he was wrong; that it was some stupid night out drinking with his brother, who had gone on and on about how everything was going to change, about "the old ball and chain", about how the sex would stop. Over the following weeks, I worked to lose the "move-in ten" pounds that I had gained, to take care of myself, to move on, to have fun again, to flirt . . . yet also to make EVERY excuse in the book to call our apartment any chance I could get. I did the "Did I leave my watch?"; and even kept up the pretense of "I need for you to NOT be there so I can pick up . . ."—it didn't matter. I just needed to stay connected to him. I knew in my heart we were meant to be together, that he just needed to work through something.

The very last phone call that I remember was when I called his parents' house. I had heard that he was at their pool—on our Sunday dinner day, without me. I called there because I had stopped at the apartment to pick something up and found a card that read "Missy" and had a phone number. Beside myself, I picked up the phone. Of course, when his mother answered, I broke down. I asked her why this was happening. And then a strange thing happened—the thing that every girlfriend hopes for and waits for: she took my side. She put Colin on the phone, and when he heard my tears, the hurt in my voice, he broke down.

"I love you, I miss you, I am so sorry, let's just not do this, I want you to move back in."

There are not many moments that you remember of those butterflies in the pit of your stomach—pure joy, pure love. I remember that feeling, and the feeling of utter relief: relief that I had not really lost him; relief that he was still going to be in my life. I had realized, while we were apart, that he was the one person I wanted to share everything with: good, bad, all of it. He was the one place I could find solace and comfort. He didn't always tell me what I wanted to hear, he told me what I needed to hear—the one thing that would always make me find comfort, or make the celebration even more joyous. He was that person for me, and I had found that out by missing him so terribly. I was going to move back in with him and never leave. I felt much better about myself, much stronger about us, much stronger about myself.

Though, the very next day, I would learn just why fate had found a chance to bring us back together when it did.

The phone rang that morning as Colin and I were lying in bed, finding solace in not missing each other, enjoying time together. To say that my stepmother and I never saw eye to eye was an understatement. I sometimes think that if we had just met, and I didn't know that she had an affair with my father, I would have liked her alright—probably would have liked her a lot, even. However, out of loyalty to my mom and out of justice, to this day I can't bring myself to like her. Why is that? She was under no obligation, my father was married, she was widowed, he should have said no, yet most of my anger was directed at her.

"I took your father to the doctor today because he ate a bad sausage," (no, seriously, that's what she said!), "and when I went to get his antibiotics I came home and found him unconscious. I called 911 and we are at the hospital right now. I think you should come."

"Did he have a heart attack?" I asked.

"They don't know," was the answer.

I put the receiver down. And because of the strange look on my face, Colin asked me what was wrong.

"My dad had a heart attack and he's not going to make it," I told him. I didn't mean to embellish, I didn't mean to lie, I didn't even think about what I was saying. I was in a trance, in shock. As I said earlier, I sometimes sense things coming long before they actually do. I knew for a long time that my father would eventually die of a heart attack. I told people in college. I even told people in high school. If it was not a self-fulfilling prophecy on my part, my father, on his, definitely talked himself into it. My father didn't have a day that he was not worried about dying—he even worried about worrying about it too much. He worried about the bills, crashing on a plane, eating too much fat, drinking too much water—he worried about everything except the things that mattered. So, when I got the call, I knew it was time. I put down the receiver, called my sister, and said the same thing to her:

"Dad had a heart attack and he is going to die."

"Is that what Brenda said?" she asked me.

"No," I replied, "that is what I know."

She picked me up and we went to the suburbs, talking the whole time about how predictable this all was. When we arrived at the emergency room, we were quickly whisked away to a "private room". Within the emergency room—you wouldn't notice it unless you have ever needed it—there is always a private room. It's where families go when they know it is serious, probably fatal, and definitely not a "quick-fix" hospital trip. That is the room.

I sat in that room as relatives quickly hustled in and out. Not my relatives, mind you.

Firstly, my father never shared his family with my sister and me. For my whole life I thought my father was probably hatched from a crazy woman and with no father. I had heard stories, all coming from my mother, about what a witch his mother was, and how he had been sent off to a military academy because his real father had just up and left. From the age of six, my father was in a military academy, going home only for Christmas and Thanksgiving. He convinced himself that everyone else was dead. He was dead to them, or them to him, but he didn't keep in touch or appear to know anyone else.

Secondly, most of those people walking in and out were probably part of the life my dad had begun without me. As here too were his "new" family, complete with stepdaughters and stepsons, children calling him "Grandpa Al"—it was all so surreal.

A woman with a clipboard came in and immediately said, "Your father is up and talking; he is going to be fine", which led right into "Does he have any religious affiliations? Any religious rituals that we should be mindful of?"

I looked over at my sister, who let this question go completely over her head. She saw it as a simple question, nothing more than information needed. However, I was able to read the true substance behind it:

"Do we need to call for last rites?"

(I guess it was a different era. True, it was only fifteen years ago, but I don't think that, even back then, anyone would get away with telling someone that a comatose patient was up and talking if that wasn't the case. Only days later did I come to find out that he did not ever regain consciousness.)

After they finally told me that it was dire and that he might not survive, there was a whole slew of people approaching me. They were bothering me because I didn't want to go back and see him. Afraid that he was going to die, they all wanted me to go see him and, in some strange ritualistic way, say goodbye. In my world and my thought process there are many things that I remain strong on. I don't have a firm religious stance, but I do believe in certain things: and I knew that, if I had something to say—something that I needed him to hear, and he was going to die—I did not need to be at his side in order for him to hear me. I knew that if his soul was going to move on, then anywhere that I was, he would be able to hear the words I needed to say.

The browbeating went on for what seemed like hours until I finally gave in. I didn't want to see him suffer. I wanted my memory of my father to be the healthy, happy, alive father who took me ice-skating and fishing. The father that danced with me at weddings, shirt soaked because there was alcohol and my father finally let loose and enjoyed himself. At weddings, he was fun. That was the Dad I wanted to remember, not someone lying on a gurney, me rushing in out of fear that what I needed to say would be to someone who was already gone. In my belief, you are never gone. You are watching over your loved ones always and forever.

At others' insistence, I walked down the long corridor of the emergency room. And just as I turned the corner to the room on the left, there lay my dad, convulsing, eyes rolling to the back of his head, foaming at the mouth.

"You forced me to see this?! *This* is what you all thought I needed to see?! What the hell is wrong with all of you?!"

That's what I remember screaming as I made my way back out into the waiting room, only to literally be caught. I fell right into Colin's arms. He had driven to see me, and with perfect timing he was there, arms open, holding me, protecting me, making it alright. That is who and what Colin is to me: my lifeline, my emergency contact, the one who makes everything worth living through.

Chapter Three

Everyone grows up thinking that their normal is everyone else's normal. Until, one day, they look around and realize that life is random. There is no order or fairness to things, and expectations aren't realistic, even if we all have them. In the end, however, if given the chance to choose someone else's experiences over your own, opting for that would be a tragedy. We all have a story to tell: that is what makes life worth living.

*

My father remained in the hospital that August for ten days. My stepmother refused to let go. She had to have three different neurologists' opinions that he was braindead before she would take him off life-support.

My sister and I always laugh about this: there are two people you never want making your health decisions if you are in a coma. The first is me; I don't believe in keeping someone's soul here if it is ready to go. The second is my mom. My mom is a completely different story. My sister and I joke that she would be saying "pull the plug" even if you were still awake. I think she just can't stand to watch someone suffer: in the same way, I suppose, as we all can't—but her faith is so strong that she is looking forward to the afterlife. When we were discussing Colin's determination to stay here, his unwillingness to give up, my mother commented:

"There has got to be something out there better than this."

"Even if there is nothing after this, which I don't believe," I answered, "that is better than this."

But my stepmother was holding on; she was not ready to watch him go.

I think about the time that I did spend alone with him, when I finally had the courage to tell him what he meant to me. Sitting there next to him, the words started pouring out, as if someone had turned on a faucet. Emotions were spewing from every direction. I was going from "You made me so mad" to "I love you" to "I hate you" to "I went into psychology to be like you". It sounds like it took hours, but it was all condensed into about ten minutes.

As I was finishing, tears streaming from my eyes—the kind of emotion that makes your palms sweat, and the crying that chokes your voice—I sat silently; and then he squeezed my hand ever so slightly. I believe that he was in between this life and the next, deciding whether he was ready to go. But in that moment, he was there, he heard me. And then there was nothing.

Three days later, my stepmother invited me to the pulling of the cord. I stepped aside to let his new family have the honors of the goodbye party. I had said my goodbyes and knew in my heart he was gone to better things and better places.

The funeral was quick. I don't remember most of it, or I have combined the memories with other funerals. I wrote a poem, which was placed on the casket. I am sure it still exists somewhere. Someday I will be cleaning out an old closet and it will resurface. That is how one's loved ones come back to remind us: through symbols of them, remembrances to keep them alive. I know someone transferred that poem for me, so I have no doubt it is somewhere. My stepmother packed up his things and gave most to her kids; didn't really offer anything to me. I don't know what, if any, of his things she has left. All I have left of him are my memories—but they are good enough, they will remain in my heart forever. Some days I love him, some days I hate him; but I will never forget him, and the older I get the more I realize that he was just a person. I needed him to be better than he was. I wanted him to be perfect. He wasn't. He was just human.

Colin and I continued with our lives. I don't think that I could have made it through that time without Colin. I was able to move forward because I felt like I was beginning a new life—a new life with Colin. When my father died, I worked for a company who had a policy of liberalism. They didn't believe in limiting the number of sick days or vacation days. They put people onto their own recognizance. Well, needless to say, the old saying is true: it just takes one to ruin it for everyone. By the time I was done with taking days to "mourn my father", the company had set a limit on personal, vacation, and sick days.

I couldn't afford any more sick days, so about five months after my father's death, when I became really sick, I couldn't take time off. That year, I had already experienced pleurisy (yes, that's right, I actually had it) and a host of other illnesses. This time however was nothing like the others. I was certain that this was it—I had cancer and I was dying. After almost a week of feeling so sick I couldn't move off the couch, and being so tired I couldn't find the energy to do much of anything, I decided that it was time to finally see a doctor. That said a lot: not only do most twenty-four-year-olds not "see doctors", but Colin was so convinced that I had an incurable illness, and so worried about me, that he accompanied me there.

On a Monday, Colin and I went to the clinic. We sat in that little room while I described my laundry list of issues, absolutely sure my time was up. The doctor I saw was part of a "teaching hospital", and on that day she had a student helping her out. He shuffled in and out the door, not asking questions, seemingly just an observer. At the beginning of the appointment, I was asked to leave urine, then she took some blood, and off the assistant went with all my bodily fluids.

The doctor was so friendly, and just the kind of doctor I needed. She was not an alarmist, and probably had discovered from our previous visits that I was somewhat of a hypochondriac. She was a teacher at the clinic, and had probably aced the part of medical school where they taught you to maintain a nondescript expression. She never looked concerned or disinterested; she had the perfect balance. She asked me myriad questions about how I was eating, and we quickly got onto the subject of how I was dealing with my father's death. I think she began to see my symptoms as generic symptoms that pointed to exhaustion and stress. She had put us both so at ease that Colin had gone into the waiting room, probably bored with the whole thing. Once the doctor didn't look grave, I suppose he thought that it must not be anything serious. The doctor came back into the tiny room and said to me that although she could not tell me for sure until the blood work was back, she was certain that whatever I was experiencing was probably just a virus. She was just going into her list of what I should do to remedy it—drink plenty of fluids, try to get rest, if I needed a doctor's note she could supply me with one—when there was a knock on the door.

The assistant, a male—I couldn't tell you what he looked like if my life depended on it—poked his head through the door. He interrupted her list of instructions to me to say, "Well, I listened to your symptoms and took the liberty of running an additional test". He looked like he was going to throw me a surprise party, and was obviously very impressed by his interference, and his findings that would have otherwise gone unnoticed. He took the paper that he was waving into the air and handed it to Dr. Meams. She took one glance at the paper, paled, and then flushed. She looked up from her paper and straight into my eyes.

"Well, Julie, I never saw this coming. I should've put it together, but with your history . . ."

I felt vomit welling up in my throat. *Here comes the death sentence*, was all I could think.

"Congratulations, you are pregnant?" she said. Her words were not a confirmation; more a question, as if she was as shocked as I was.

I sat speechless. I don't remember being excited. I don't remember being sad or worried. I don't remember feeling much of anything. It was as if the words reached me and then just bounced off and trailed onto the floor. Instantly I was in an alternate universe. Then I quickly panicked at worrying about telling Colin—how on earth was I going to tell Colin?! Part of me wished he had stayed in the room so that I didn't have to break the news to him. The other part of me was so glad that he was not there, because I felt like I needed to get my bearings.

"Julie, Julie . . . are you going to be okay? You look like you're going to pass out . . . why don't you just sit for a while?"

"No, I'm fine," I uttered, as I regained my balance, swallowing hard.

"Do you want me to come with you while you tell your boyfriend?" She was keenly aware of the situation I was about to face and knew all too well that not only was this a shock to my system, but there was someone in the waiting room who was about to hear something that would forever alter his life.

"No, I'll be fine."

Still in shock, I opened the door and walked through. I paused very briefly in the hallway, brushed off my pants as if I had gotten dust or soot on them, trying to remove the stain of the situation that I had just come from—almost like, if I looked put back together, then I would be so. I steadied my gait and made an unconscious agreement with myself that I was going to walk straight up to Colin, maintain my composure, and just tell him, without crying or hysterics. As I joined Colin, he looked at me. From the look on my face—I didn't even have to say "Let's go"—he just jumped up, like I had some tractor beam that propelled him from his seat.

I can't honestly say that it was that I felt comfortable in falling apart, or whether it was out of sheer guilt. I can remember looking into his blue eyes and thinking, *How can I take his youth? How can I end his boyishness in this very moment? He is going to hate me forever.* We walked briskly to the elevator: Colin silent, reaching for my hand, trying desperately to get a feel for what had happened in those brief moments he was not there. Maybe questioning what could have gone so terribly wrong in a matter of minutes. Maybe feeling guilty for not staying with me. He didn't question me, or speak, since I was avoiding his gaze. Awaiting the elevator, he pressed the down button and we stood silent for what seemed like hours. I began to shake, as if keeping it inside and keeping it to myself might actually make me explode. By this point tears were coming: at first trickling, and now falling rapidly as I was trying to hide them. I was wiping them: first from the corner of my eyes, as if I could stop them from coming; then had resorted to my sleeve; and now fluids were flowing from my nose and I was making those hiccup noises you make when you are trying hard not to cry, which never works out. Colin stood terrified.

The elevator finally arrived at our floor, and in my hurry to get in it I almost knocked over the three people that were attempting to exit. As we entered the elevator, Colin looked at me with a terror I have only seen a couple times in our lifetime together. I had tears streaming down my eyes and ten years of disbelief about what my life had in store for me, shot to hell.

"Oh my God, are you really dying?" he asked.

"No. I'm pregnant," I replied, just as the elevator doors closed in front of my eyes and the world as I had known it closed along with it.

Somewhere along my journey into womanhood I had decided that children were not on the cards for me. It wasn't that I didn't want them—just the opposite; that's all I wanted. But, in some old Irish

Catholic way, I was somehow sacrificing myself to be childless long before a decision of fates was truly made. My impression was somewhat based on fact. My medical history was marred with hormonal issues, so I thought it was clear that I was to live a life without children. Not only did I not take precautions, but I had always assured Colin that there really was no reason to. But God had a different plan—He always does.

And so when I found out, once the shock hard worn off, I was elated. The one thing that I wanted in my life that I was sure I would never have: it was here in front of me, a gift.

That is the way that I saw this pregnancy: it was a gift. All those years of feeling like it would never happen, all those years of crying that I would be without children, all of it began to fade away. The fear of having this child, the fear of pregnancy, gave way to the realization that I was going to have the one thing that I had always wanted.

Unfortunately, Colin did not feel the same way. It wasn't that he didn't want children—quite the contrary. He was just being realistic and fearing the responsibility. I have come to realize over the years that most guys have the same response to pregnancy. The moment they hear that they are going to have a child, one thing runs through their heads. Money. All they can concentrate on is, how will they afford a child? Since Colin was still clerking down at the Board of Trade, making $5 an hour, well, he was not ready for the responsibility of affording a child. He was emotionally ready—he probably had been from birth!—but he was not financially ready, and it scared him more than anything.

So he retreated, he shut me out, he sulked, so angry was he to be in this position. I sat on the outside, not knowing what to do;

not knowing what was going to undo what I had done; feeling so responsible for his unhappiness, but feeling happiness myself—so conflicted.

Chapter Four

I walk down this long corridor out of the chemo land fog, not realizing that the sky has opened up and it is sunny. Outside in the world around us it is sunny. In here it is always dark. In here rain is always pending.

*

It was a tough couple of months spent readjusting my thinking on life, and redefining my path and goals. I knew that I was going to keep the baby. There was never a question in my mind, as I told my sister and my mom. But to Colin, I said that there was a choice. I told him that it was his decision. In my twenty-four-year-old's brain, I believed that if I didn't give him the choice, that if I didn't allow him to come to the decision on his own, he would always end up resenting me and the baby. So I played along with him. I said that I would end the pregnancy if that was what he wanted. I even made the appointment. But I knew that that was never in my heart. I wanted this baby more than anything, and if he was not going to come around—well then, I would have this baby all on my own. I also knew in Colin's soul that he wanted his baby too. When I finally went in for the ultrasound and saw the heartbeat, I decided that I was no longer playing games. One night after many tears were shed—my side being presented, then his—he looked at me and said, "Let's go get dessert". So off we went to the Golden Apple. It was a place we frequented—though never sober, and never before three a.m. We sat quietly in a booth, ordered our sundaes, and with the fifth bite he took, he looked at me and said, "So we're going to do this, huh?" Then nothing but silence again.

Colin and I were struggling with leaving our immaturity behind. In some small town we might have been at a ripe old age to have children, but in downtown Chicago we were babies who were too selfish to look after even ourselves. The friends that we had spent so many years partying with? Well, they carried on partying. It was hard to relearn how to be a person. We were still in that same apartment, still with the same friends, still the same couple—but everything in our lives was different. I continued to work, while Colin became more serious about his. He started really making some money, feeling confident, feeling more secure in his ability and his skills to really make a good living to support us.

One day Colin called and was all excited about getting some tickets to watch the Cubs game. Mind you, the very last thing that I wanted to do was to go to a Cubs game. Cubs games for me were only fun when I was half in the bag, didn't really care about the game, and didn't really care who was winning; but I knew that if I didn't at least try to regain some semblance of our old relationship, he might give up all together. I agreed to leave work "sick" and head to the game with him. It was a hot day, in the eighties, and to say that the maternity wear in the nineteen nineties was not so attractive was an understatement. I had on a red-and-white-checkered jumpsuit: something that looked like it belonged more on an Italian restaurant table than on a large pregnant woman.

He swung close by my office to pick me up and off we headed. When we arrived at the stadium, the tickets were right smack-dab in the middle of the bleachers. The bleachers are the most fun of the seats for sure, but only for those who want to go topless, to drink lots, to show off their tube tops and rock-solid abs. We took our seats behind the bachelorette party in full swing next to the marine section, where they were all topless and flirting with each other, beer spilling everywhere. I began to sweat, not just a little, but profusely. For anyone who has been pregnant before, your body temperature is so high that just the slightest change in temperature can send you into a complete meltdown.

I sat in those bleachers watching all the fun, all the beautiful and attractive people our age, all the drinks flowing; trying so hard to not look miserable, trying so hard to be a good sport, to show Colin that I was the same girl. I wanted him to see that I could still be fun, that things were not all that different or gone forever, sweat pouring from my face.

He finally looked over at me and literally blurted out "Oh my God Julie . . . Are you okay?" I literally was melting. "Not really," was all I could manage to answer, and as I was feverishly wiping the sweat from my brow it was streaming down my face, soaking my awful outfit. He stood, extended his arm for me to grab onto, and began to make his way out of the bleachers and down the stairs, rescuing me from my obvious misery. Sweat was coming from every part of my body, but I was trying so hard to be fun, so hard to be pretty. I was neither. I avoided his gaze as we made our way through the crowd: him grabbing for my hand, me avoiding the grip with sweaty hands that I needed free in order to continually swipe my forehead. We stood on the corner attempting to get a cab. Here I finally raised my eyes just carefully enough to get a glimpse of him looking back at me. He had a look of pity, but it was softened by a look of sheer love and sympathy; for as much as I was trying to be the person I was previous to the pregnancy, he was trying to pretend I was that person as well— but not for himself, for me. He could see my obvious discomfort and my desperate attempt to hold on to who I was, hold on to who we were as people, as a couple. He sensed that I needed to be in denial. I needed him to be in denial as well.

After Jake, our first son, was born, I decided to return to graduate school, knowing realistically that I couldn't continue to work the hours that I had. With me not in employment, we couldn't afford to maintain our lifestyle, and so when my mom offered to let us move into her rental in the suburbs we quickly took it— heading back to the town where we had met and grown up in. My mother made us the offer that, instead of renting her home, we could do a wrap-around mortgage—basically a rent-to-buy option. Before we had even signed the papers, we ripped out walls, sledgehammered drywall, tore up flooring, took down ceilings: all before even giving my mother a dime. Needless to say she was a nervous wreck, though she tried to keep it to herself.

While we were tearing the house apart, we needed a place to stay. Colin's parents, who lived in more of an estate than a home, offered us their coach house, which was a one-bedroom, one-bath cottage, located just outside of the pool area.

So we lived in that cottage. It was mostly Jake and I alone while Colin was at work. Meanwhile I had scheduled it so I only had to attend graduate school two days a week.

The trek to school was a whole-day event. I was getting my degree in public health (which I fondly explained was really "1001 things that will kill you that you can't do anything about"). I was commuting downtown to the University of Illinois, which was in the worst area of the city. The building that housed my program was located right in the middle of a triangle that consisted of the Cook County Hospital, the Cook County Juvenile Court, and the WIC program food mart. The buildings were all dilapidated, rat-infested, and most assuredly plagued by asbestos and any other harmful material that time could have invented. There were little police-call buttons on the sidewalk in between the buildings, which were supposed to lend comfort to those of us who attended. (It didn't.) That winter, there had been several occurrences of random sexual assaults within the block where I attended classes. I tried to schedule only day classes, but some were only offered at night, which ended up making me a nervous wreck. I would dread going downtown, and would park my car and literally run to the buildings where I was supposed to be.

I spent my weekdays trying to finish up my master's as quickly as I could, and we spent our nights and weekends knocking out walls and tearing out ceilings in a house we hadn't paid a dime on.

Luckily, Colin was not like me: he finished what he started. He believed in doing one thing at a time and doing it well, finishing one project before moving on to the next. And so after a year of working on our home, the job was finally done. We had taken a three-bedroom home and made it into a single-room space—open floor plan, yet no separate bedroom for us. We had not prioritized a bedroom for us. We knew we were not done building our dream, and decided to move in, begin our life, and make the rest up as we went along.

I continued finishing up my master's, but that novelty wore off as soon as we no longer needed the financial aid. Colin was really figuring out the whole trading thing and starting to make a living at it. Since all I ever wanted to do was to stay home, I did odds and ends. Jake had just started preschool, and he was completely and utterly not okay with it, but probably more so because I was not okay with it. I needed him just as much—if not more—than he needed me. I would try to drop him off and the tears would start; the grabbing of my legs; the "don't go"s and "don't leave me"s; and, by the time it was over, he was in the car on the way home with me again. Yes, it was obsessive and crazy, probably not mentally healthy, but it worked for me.

*

If there is one thing I've been able to do it's to never look back and regret a choice that I have made. I don't know if it is arrogance, an assuredness, or just the understanding that truly everything does happen for a reason. There is not one single thing that we do in our lives that doesn't affect everything around it. Good or bad, every choice, every decision is like a crossroads that we choose for some means to an end.

*

Once we moved into the house, in a display of my obsessive need for upheaval I decided Jake needed a sibling. That became my new mission. The longing to have another child, to experience the joy that I felt with Jake, was ingrained into my soul. Colin was not happy—he thought (rightly so) that we had enough going on, but I was determined and had one thing now to accomplish. I wanted so badly to be pregnant again.

But while the first one came so easily, number two did not.

Chapter Five

As you sit in the waiting area, you can't help but look around, comparing the misfortunes of others to your own. You feel guiltily elated but instantly remorseful when you see someone worse off than you, and you feel instantly hopeful when the next person called up for the chair looks like they must have been the sick person's driver rather than the sick person themselves. But on rare occasions like today, you feel a weird combo of both blessed and saddened beyond words.

    I sat typing away on my BlackBerry while two teenage girls in the waiting room chairs next to me were giggling, as if they were in line to get their driver's licenses. As I looked at them I realized this seemingly healthy teenage girl who was a robust beaming blonde had an IV line—an IV line to receive the same poison as everyone else around me. I always considered Colin way too young to be sick, but as I looked over at this girl, who has not yet experienced so much of what life has to offer, I found myself silently praying for an "easy" cancer for her. As if I'm ordering off a cancer menu, I am asking for her to have a plate of leukemia or lymphoma. I am praying it is not our fate.

*

Over the next two years, I was obsessed with having another child. And in those two years, I would have two early miscarriages. The first came early on. Although I had only just found out that I was pregnant, as any woman who has experienced a miscarriage can tell you, the minute you get a positive result, you've already thought about what college they are going to. The second was on my birthday. I had started having cramps and spotting during the day, so I was nervous yet still hopeful. I had resigned myself to wearing an old silver cross that my mother had given me—I thought now was the time to enlist God. I called the doctor, waited for Colin to come home from work, and on 9 March they squeezed me in for the very last appointment for the day. We sat in the waiting room, both of us joking yet tense. *Surely*, I thought, *this won't be anything but good news, on my birthday*. But I knew in my heart it wasn't. We were brought into the room, the exam started, and as I watched the ultrasound technician's face I knew that my worst fears were being realized.

"I am so sorry to tell you this, but I can't find a heartbeat." She touched my knee and then she headed towards the door. "I'll have the doctor come in and talk with you." That was all she said as she exited the room.

Colin and I stood speechless. After my father passed away, I went through a tiny box filled with his belongings. He kept his past to himself, so it was full of with trinkets and things and people I didn't know or recognize. He was a very religious man, and among his valuables there was a necklace with a charm of St. Mary. The moment I saw it, I felt like it was special to him; and it struck me that, if it meant something to him, it meant something to me. When I became pregnant, for some reason I started wearing it—almost as if I felt it had some protective properties; or maybe it gave me some comfort in thinking I was connected to him with it and that he was looking over me, him protecting me. In that moment, I pulled the necklace off. I wrestled with myself, as all I wanted to do was to take it and throw it across the room. The God that I knew, the God that I had grown up with . . . at that very moment, He no longer existed; He was dead to me. I sat with that cross in my hand, hating God, cursing Him, but I couldn't bring myself to throw it. I *could* shut the door to my faith in that moment. However, I just wanted to shelf it. I handed the necklace to Colin. Poor Colin stood next to me. I was so angry that I couldn't even muster tears; so defiantly angry was I that I was not going to give God the satisfaction of crying.

In came the doctor. I don't remember her apologizing for our loss or anything to that effect. Instead what she said was:

"Because you are so far along, I think that we have to schedule a D&C to remove the material."

"Can't I just wait? Won't it just come out on its own?"

"I'm afraid not, so we will get you in hopefully this week. I can't call anyone tonight; it's too late. But call here in the morning and we'll figure something out." That was all she said. Then she turned and left me and Colin—bewildered, sitting quietly in this room, mourning, devastated.

I am sure Colin had wanted to come to my aid, but, looking at the fury in my eyes, he realized that now was not the time. He knew me well enough and had seen me face enough tough situations to know it was best to just let the emotion run its course. But I misread it as him not caring. In my selfish immaturity, I thought that I was the only one who lost something in that room—and on my birthday. There was not an ounce of me that felt Colin was sad or was mourning. In fact, I immediately said, "I was the one that wanted this baby; you are probably happy".

When we got home, I walked in the door, went immediately up to my bedroom, and lay there in the quiet, just sobbing. Colin was downstairs, watching TV and hoping to wait out the storm of my anger. I got up after about an hour and went down to him.

"You don't care, do you? You don't care that I lost this baby. You're even happy—look at you! You just don't even give a shit, do you?"

I'd come up behind Colin, flinging those words at him like they were rocks.

"Of course I care, Jules. I love you, I loved this baby too; I wanted this baby, I was excited. I just don't know what to say to you. I don't know how to make this okay for you. I feel like I am walking on a landmine with anything I say, so I am just trying to be quiet, to let you work through it. What do you need me to say? What do you want me to say?"

That was the point where my anger started to fade away and I let my guard down. I sat down next to him, and there was finally a flash of relief.

"You know, we can try again," he began. "This is a good sign; we know you can have another baby. I know this is hard, but we will try again, and we will have another baby," he said, as I folded into him. For the first time, probably in my whole life, I felt like I was right where I belonged and with exactly who I belonged with.

The doctor's office called the next day and I was scheduled for surgery the day after. I stayed in bed that entire day with the covers pulled up. Now I was terrified that something would happen to me. I thought about Jake being motherless should I not make it through the surgery, and the unfairness of the whole situation just seemed to snowball. This meant that, on the following day, when we headed off for surgery, I was a mess. I couldn't stop crying. I couldn't even reply to their questions at the office, so Colin had to step in and answer. Until they were finally able to put me under to finish the procedure, I am sure that I made a lot of already anxious patients even more so.

When I woke up, they asked me if I would like to have the remains buried. Honestly, I think I said, "No, it wasn't anything but tissue". I needed to have coldness in my heart if I was to survive.

"Yes, I think we should," came the voice from beside me.

It was about the only thing that I can recall Colin voicing any opinion on. And so they handed me some literature and a birth certificate and told me where the fetus was to be buried. It is all still somewhere in my basement. I could never find it in me to look at any of it, but it is there: among the old IRS forms and tax receipts. I needed to put it away—out of sight, out of mind. Now, as I think about it, I am both sad and hopeful that Colin might soon able to meet that little soul we only had in our lives a couple of weeks.

After healing (at least physically), I found out that August that we were hoping to expect our second child on 15 May the following year. I was elated, yet completely terrified at the same time.

One wrong move . . . I thought. Too much exertion, too much caffeine, secondhand smoke, microwaved food: it all became my enemy. My new best friend were those newfangled antibacterial products, which were exploding at the time thanks to a marketing campaign on crack. I started to put distance between me and Jake during that time. When he was four, we went to movies together, we hung out and went to plays, had lunch together, and he was my best friend. But at the same time, he became in my eyes a walking death germ. Everything that he touched might be tainted with some form of disease that would kill the new baby growing inside of me.

I still feel so sad to this day when he won't tell me that he is sick. I once thought he didn't tell me because that was who he was—controlled, not wanting a fuss—but I now see it was years of conditioning. You see, well before Taytem (the girl I wanted to put in a bubble) came along, there had been the endless precious pregnancies. As soon as Jake would utter the word "sick", or even indicate that he was not feeling well, he would be sequestered to his room, becoming a prisoner. There was no holding, soothing, coddling, as there had been pre-miscarriages. There was just loneliness and meals left at the door. There was probably no rhyme or reason for him to my sudden aloofness and withdrawal. I was so terrified that an illness would take this baby too that I really distanced myself from him.

*

All these years later, I am still fighting to make that right, to reconnect what I lost with him: mostly the trust of unconditional love, which most assuredly felt very conditional at the time. There are many, many regrets I have about how I have conducted myself and how I have treated others, but the way I treated my four-year-old—who had no idea what he had done wrong—that is the top of my list.

Chapter Six

Just as I had distanced myself from my four-year-old in an attempt to save pregnancies I had no control over, seven years later I am doing the same thing to Colin. My inability to hug Colin through everything is just a carryover of my inability to deal with loss and sadness; my repeat behavior like déjà vu.

Tayt's pregnancy, as hard as it might be to accept, was meant to happen the way that it did, whether or not I distanced and protected myself. Looking back, I don't think at that time I knew or understood what a true miracle it was. I think that on a daily basis; plus, when something happens with her, the miracle is made even more vivid. Like when I recently attended a meeting at her school. They began by telling me that she would never learn. They told me she was incapable of learning, and not only was she not good enough to be in the first grade, but that she should join others "like her" at a special school.

Tears began streaming from my eyes, but not because I was sad at what they were telling me. They weren't telling me anything about her that I didn't already know. I knew she was going to have a hard time reading, and that her academic performance was never going to be "normal", but I also knew that it didn't matter. I sat there listening to their droning voices, anger growing inside me as the pictures of what Tayt had been through flashed across my consciousness. My heart was literally screaming at them, *How dare you?! Do you have ANY idea what this little soul, what her father, what I have been through to get her to where she is?! Do you have any idea about the little soul that lives within her?! She might not be able to read or to remember her alphabet, but I bet she remembers every one of your names. She remembers when someone makes fun of her, or when someone makes her feel stupid. If she is so incapable of learning, how come she has learned to not trust anyone like you as you are sitting here judging her?!*

Halfway through the meeting, with me in tears, I excused myself and said that I was expected elsewhere. I took off out the door. The last thing I heard was something about, "It's up to you; think about it. It's for her own good to be with other children like her".

Trust me when I say there is NO ONE "like" Taytem. There never has been, and there never will be. So whatever these children were like, they were *not* like Taytem—nor would they ever be. I just pray that, in my attempts to always save Taytem, I haven't lost the people who also needed me along the way.

*

I remember the first ultrasound. When they found a heartbeat, they proudly announced, "You are six weeks pregnant". And then again two weeks later, the heartbeat and the announcement, "You are six weeks pregnant". And then again another two weeks after. It was like

I was stuck in the Ben Murray movie *Groundhog Day*, wherein they kept informing me I was six weeks pregnant. When I insisted that they were now telling me that I gotten pregnant *four weeks after* I was initially told I was pregnant, they shrugged it off as bad calculations and just changed my due date.

That is how that pregnancy went: a million recantations, miscalculations, misstatements, and misdiagnoses rolled into nine months of neuroses. I began bleeding—not a lot, but enough to send up a red flag—and that day (when we went in for my fifth of *forty-seven* ultrasounds), I was told that there was a placental tear in the amniotic sac and there was a fifty-fifty chance of losing the pregnancy.

I would be in bed for weeks on end, trying to save a pregnancy that was destined to unfold the way it was supposed to, regardless of my actions. Bedrest wouldn't have saved any of the previous pregnancies, but I was told this time it would. And this time *would* be different. If I let that tear heal, Tayt would be saved and she would live.

After following the doctor's orders, the bleeding stopped, and at the next ultrasound the tear had repaired itself. Tayt had grown the amount she should have, her heartbeat resounded clearly, and we thought that the worst was over. I was going to get to keep her. I was carefully monitored from that moment on. I had an ultrasound literally every week, and there was a sick feeling that would ensue prior to each scan. That measurement became more a measurement of her odds of making it.

Anytime I thought we were in the clear and that the pregnancy was going to be alright, the phone would ring and there was some new test telling us that Tayt was not "doing well", although no one could tell us what was going on. Her growth was definitely varied, but, with the exception of that, all was fine. Anatomically she was perfect. Petite and proportionately tiny, but perfect. I remember I was doing something in the kitchen—probably dishes from breakfast—right after Jake had just gone off to school. I was in my fifteenth week at that time, which was when my doctor called to let me know that the fetal testing that I had done indicated it was extremely likely that Tayt had Trisomy 18: a third eighteenth chromosome. She told me that the elevated blood levels of the test had indicated that there was a high likelihood that Tayt was not going to make it to birth—or, if she did, the three number 18 chromosomes meant she would be born yet would die painfully and most assuredly within the first year of life.

I had always told myself that I was incapable of terminating a pregnancy, so I waited. In my mind, I needed proof: some tangible evidence of faulty wiring. I needed a cleft palate, I needed a clubfoot, I needed clubbed hands.

While this pregnancy was consuming our lives, we were also knee-deep in opening a restaurant. As I said, we had moved back to "Boringtown", as we fondly named it, and we planned along with some friends to open a hometown restaurant bar named after our high-school mascot. Looking back, it was our immersion into this project that got me through. It was the distraction that took away from the gravity of the situation, and was the sheer bustle that allowed me to function on autopilot. Eventually, though, when the pregnancy started to kick into high gear and things went south, we had to sell our part of the ownership. I didn't miss it, yet I think Colin missed a place to find some breathing room from the seriousness of the confines of our home.

Chapter Seven

As I sit here with Colin, a random nurse starts asking basic questions. They quickly turn into a discussion of Tayt, her trach, her therapy, the proverbial "Wow, you guys have been through so much". Although it can sometimes be very therapeutic to talk about the journey Colin and I have been on, sometimes it is overwhelming as well. Years ago I tried to avoid Tayt's story. My wish is to someday tell it without the hurt and anger: to simply tell of the miraculous nature of her being.

*

As anyone who has ever gotten potentially drastic life-changing test results from a doctor knows, it always comes on a Friday. That means you are given an appetizer of terrible news, though no entrée to follow it up—for what feels like a long time. That is what that weekend was like: web searches, Googling "Trisomy 18" and what it meant. What it meant was that Tayt would either come out completely incapable of life, but could wait around to suffer for a couple of months, unresponsive, only to die slowly and in pain—or, she could be born one hundred percent normal. I sat on this information for months. I was told that there really was nothing more we could do unless we did an amniocentesis. I couldn't handle that; the odds of the baby surviving were too low, especially if she was weak anyway. So instead we opted to do a more intricate ultrasound.

I was told that if she did indeed have Trisomy 18, it would be horrible. There would be telltale markings on the fetus that would indicate that she had it. She would have the cleft palate, the clubfoot, the clubbed hands. There were actually six such markers. So, on that fateful day in my sixteenth week, Colin and I sat with an ultrasound technician as she did a full check to look for the markers. As the end of the exam, we were told that Tayt exhibited none of them. Not only did she exhibit no Trisomy 18, but also none of the Down's Syndrome traits, which could equally have explained the blood levels. It was then that we were told we were expecting a girl. After seeing her, after seeing her heartbeat, her profile, her sucking her thumb, my resolve to have her at ANY cost only deepened.

Although the thought that she had some sort of chromosomal issue was somewhat put on the back burner unless I did an amniocentesis, and therefore it could not be confirmed, the issue remained that she still failed to grow the way she should. At twenty-one weeks, knowing the risks involved, I gave in and agreed to have an amniocentesis done. The questioning was too much, and the stress of not knowing was beginning to take its toll. On a cold snowy day, we waited in the specialist's office to be called to have the needle injected into my belly. First though, we went in to see the fetal diagnostic specialist. (There are entire fields of medicine that just diagnose problems—or lack thereof.) The doctor who was doing the ultrasound was supposed to be the best.

He sat with us that day for what seemed like an eternity: nitpicking, looking over and over for the same markers that had been looked for before; and, come the end, he had found no evidence either. He told us that he had been ninety-nine-point-nine percent right throughout his career, and although one false diagnosis had been missed, in his opinion this was definitely NOT a chromosomal issue. He did though suggest that we have the amnio, since it was the only way to be sure.

When the amnio was over and we were on the road, I fretted all the way home about losing her and how I would live with the guilt of needing certainty and not believing in fate. Each bump of the Jeep meant certain puncturing of the amniotic fluid and death for Tayt. I was told that there would be some "rapid" results in five days, and full results within a couple of weeks. Now I just needed to focus on the restaurant and not think about the result—as if that were possible. I spent the rest of that day and the next in bed, and, after that, when I showed no signs that the procedure had done any damage, I trudged on with my daily routine.

Chapter Eight

As we sit on chemoday I call home to check on my fast-approaching-adolescent son. I tell him dress warm because he is going snow tubing. I go through my mental gathering of his items. "Make sure they are dry." "Don't forget your face mask." Tell him where to find everything. Piece it all together for him, to ease my guilt of being absent so many times physically as well as mentally. So many times he's been left to fend for himself—me absent, taking care of someone or something else. How many nights my last thought as my head has hit the bed is *Tomorrow I will spend more time with Jake. Tomorrow I will pay him more attention.* But realistically he is growing, and growing away from me, and so the guilt grows.

"Have fun be safe I love you."

Silence, and then an "Okay bye".

*

Five days later I received a call: her chromosomes came back completely normal. Certainly this was the news that I had been waiting for. Now there was no turning back. So what if she wasn't growing? It was something else wrong with her then. When she came out, she would gain the size, the strength, the health that she was lacking in the womb. She would come out perfect, normal and healthy. For the first time in so long that I can't even give a timeline, I exhaled. I don't think I knew that I wasn't breathing, sleeping, living. I was waiting—I was waiting to celebrate this pregnancy. At twenty-two weeks we were now just going to monitor, cross our fingers that the placenta would get her through the next couple of weeks, and would go in for ultrasounds and non-stress tests from that point, until we decided to deliver her.

I went into my regular OB-GYN first on a weekly basis, then every other day; I had scheduled appointments with the specialists group once a month. At twenty-three weeks I went in to have one of many, many ultrasounds. Colin, who had already taken way too much time off to soothe my angst, was not able to come, so I asked my mother-in-law—though not because I needed her for comfort. I asked her because I thought it would be a cool experience for her to see the scan and get a glimpse of her first granddaughter.

Once the ultrasound ended, a female doctor new to the specialists group was the one who received the report. We were in a room smaller than my bathroom, a makeshift office the group rented out as a satellite, with her sitting across from me behind a tiny desk. I don't remember her introducing herself, or saying *anything* to me at that, before she gave me the news that her professional opinion was that Tayt had a syndrome whereby she didn't have the ability to swallow. When I asked what that meant, I was told that she would come out and not be able to take her first breath, and that she would die as she was unable to take in air. The look on my mother-in-law's face was one of sheer terror. I felt the world crashing in on me once again. Just two short weeks ago we were told with ninety-nine-point-nine-percent surety that she was okay. Now we were back revisiting the potential that there was something unfixable with my baby. Although I was used to the roller coaster ride, Diana had just hopped on and was not enjoying the twists and turns.

I went home and waited again for my doctor to call. When she called me, she sounded furious. I had seen a specialist new to the neonatal practice. And, in that new colleague's opinion, Tayt was going to die. Yet I was told by my doctor not to listen to her. I was told that this specialist had had no right to make that definitive decision. What I wasn't told was that the new specialist was wrong.

After many more ultrasounds, I was starting to show signs that I wasn't going to make it to my due date. The stress was not only doing me harm, they feared it was hurting both of us.

They wanted me to come in and deliver Tayt on a Wednesday at nine a.m. I went in; she was thirty-four weeks at the time and weighed just three pounds (or so they thought). The day before I was told that they were going to run a test to make sure that her lungs were developed enough. So I was given yet another amniocentesis, right there in the office (and this time definitely more painful). Yet as I left in tears, I found some solace in the fact that this was all going to be over. Tomorrow was the day: Tayt was coming out; win, lose, or draw. She was either going to breathe or not, but she would be here.

We had hidden the pregnancy to the extent that most of our friends had no idea that I was even expecting. I hid it; I didn't want to talk about it; I denied it; I pretended that I wasn't. But as much as

I tried to deny her existence—as much as I tried to convince myself that I wasn't attached—I was more attached than I had been to any other pregnancy. I had invested more emotion, worry, and fretting in this little life than I had probably in anything else I could remember. The energy, the devastation, and the elation—it was all going to end tomorrow. If she died I would be devastated, no doubt, but it would be over.

The next day, Colin and I took off for the hospital. There, I got undressed and had the IVs hooked up. My regular doctor said, "I'm sure that her lungs will be fine and we are far enough along at this point". I lay in bed, just waiting to get the process going. About forty-five minutes after admission, papers were filled out and butterflies were in my stomach. The nurse came in to tell me that there was a call for me on the phone. I picked up the receiver to hear my regular doctor, the one I trusted most, say, "Her lungs are premature. We can't do this today. We are going to give you some steroids and try to get her lungs to mature over the next seventy-two hours and try again". I got dressed slowly, crying the whole time. This was not the day to find out. Bitterly, I remember thinking, *If she is going to die anyway, what is the point of all of this?*

Three days came and went and I returned to the hospital. As if it was routine, I got undressed, hoping they would pull the trigger this time, yet scared to death regardless of whether they would or wouldn't. To this day, I often wonder whether if Tayt had had a couple more weeks, could she have had the weight, the strength, the maturity, to not have all the medical tribulations that she has endured? If I had been able to withstand more—suck it up, take it in stride, not fall apart—would they have waited those crucial four more weeks?

Or, if they had waited another couple of days, would she have died in utero as they predicted?

This time was it. I received no last-minute calls. They hooked up the IV; they started the oxytocin; and it was go time. No turning back. At three p.m. on a Friday they broke Tayt's bag . . .

*

. . . and that was the catalyst for seven years of what some might call bad luck, leading to me sitting in this cancer ward hell, waiting on Colin's poison.

*

Once they broke the bag it kicked everything into high gear. After about ten minutes, Tayt's heart rate kept crashing. At first they tried to convince me it would be alright, and for the next ten minutes they attempted to stabilize her heart rate. They had me move from my right side to my left. Each time it would be okay at first, and then pretty quickly she would start crashing again. I think they realized that they needed to just get her out of whatever hell she was living in. It was time that we all got to meet Tayt. She was ready to enter the world.

At that point, they started prepping me for a C-section. I don't really remember much other than people running around frantically, gurneys, bright lights—quite a different scenario from when I'd had Jake four years earlier. Colin sat by my side throughout it all. He kept me steady. He had such a comforting look in his eyes that he was able to calm me; to let me know that, whatever we were about to face, we were going to do it together. That I was not alone in this. I would never be alone in any of it.

Finally, I heard someone say, "It's a girl", and I heard my baby cry. Yes, she took her first breath, and her second, possibly her third. I looked at Colin, who was already out of his seat, waiting to see his eyes telling me that it was alright—that she had ten fingers, ten toes, that she was alive—and then came a noise. This noise is burned into my soul. They called it stridor. Along with the strained breathing noise I heard the doctor call out "Her umbilical cord is wrapped around her neck, and we're having a hard time oxygenating her. She's crashing". The calmness of the birth turned once more to frantic running around. The doctors went from warming Tayt under the lights to whisking her away quickly.

Later, Colin came to my room, where I had a morphine pump hooked up to me. "They're going to take her to Children's Hospital," he told me. "I'm going to go with her. I can't go in the ambulance, so I am going to meet her downtown. I am so sorry that I am leaving you here. I just need to go with her to make sure that someone is."

"Of course," I replied, still not even fully aware of what was going on. I can't imagine how it must have felt for Colin having to make the decision to leave me there, lying in a hospital bed, and to head into the unknown without me. He most certainly knew he was going to have to carry the burden of what was going on with her, the decisions of what to do with her. I was in my own little world and, God love Colin, he let me stay there. They had whisked her away to the neonatal intensive care unit (NICU), and I was told that they were prepping her for transfer. They would be sending her to a larger hospital that was more equipped to handle a baby as "sick" as Tayt.

Taytem was born with pulmonary hypertension. You know, all these years later, I am still not quite sure what that means, or how that relates to any other medical conditions. All I knew was that they said she couldn't breathe on her own, and that she needed *more*—she needed more specialists, and the kind of help that the current hospital could not supply. They had transferred me to the post-op room, started my morphine drip, and separated us indefinitely.

After hours of "prepping" her—which really came down to resuscitating her every time in order to keep her alive—they were ready for the transfer. My doctor insisted that they get me a wheelchair and bring me down to see her before she set off. An argument ensued, with the resident insisting I could go into shock and die, but Riles was not giving in. She knew me well enough to know that I would have preferred death over not ever seeing the daughter whom, unbeknownst to me, everyone believed would not make it through the evening. She put me into a wheelchair and got me down to the NICU as they were "bagging" her, which equated to pumping oxygen through a bag on an ongoing basis and getting her ready for transport. I grabbed on to her tiny, tiny finger, glaring at the tubes (so many tubes), ports, IVs, breathing apparatus. She was barely the size of my palm. Weighing only three pounds, they had her drugged into a coma to keep her from touching anything, from trying to fight, from trying to live on her own; they had used medication to literally paralyze her. As I was wheeled away, I saw the tag on her transport incubator, which simply read "baby girl Barth". That name would stick. For months on end, she would only be known as "baby girl Barth".

Colin headed out after the transport ambulance and was told to take his time, because it was going to be a long night. I had no idea at the time that they were telling him she probably would not make it. As I sat there back at the hospital, dawn began to break on a new day. There is a mandatory seventy-two-hour hold after a C-section, but since they thought she was going to die, the doctors let me go after twenty-four.

After getting all my things together, my mother drove like a madwoman up to the front and frantically placed me in her car. Within forty-five minutes we were at Children's Hospital in Chicago. I walked through the doors of the hospital, not realizing that soon it would become my home. I had no idea that I would pass through that check-out station every day to grab my security tag, each time giving them a look that said, "Really? Everyone here knows me; is this really necessary?" It was simultaneously cold and sterile and dirty. An older woman was at the front booth, and she was completely incapable of understanding the simplest of names. Names like Smith or Jones were unrecognizable to her. As many times as I saw her over the next four months and expected her to remember my face, she never did. I gathered up my visitor's pass, which would soon be like a badge to enter work, and followed the red line to the elevators that would take me up to see a daughter I had not really had the opportunity to meet.

At the entrance of the ward there was a desk set up to check your tag. The employee there did get to know me, and wouldn't even glance up whenever I would walk by. She had almost learned my gait; the shuffle of my shoes must have been distinctive enough for her (and everyone else) to know to just ignore me. But since this was my initial induction into the NICU, she asked my name and pointed to a nurse who then escorted me into a large room, wherein Colin was sitting and waiting for me. We had been unable to talk on the phone because Colin had been glued here, by Tayt's side, since her arrival. He had not left her except to shower in the family section and return.

There were four incubators around the room, each with their own watchdog nurse and monitors blipping and beating, sometimes in unison. And when one of their four inhabitants' machines strayed from the unison, cacophony ensued. Someone would rush over and do something: a flip, a shot, a suction, a med. Something to bring the room's alerts back to synchronicity. Colin was seated in an office chair. In true Colin fashion, he had his elbows over the chair, a cup of ice in his hand, as he steadily watched the numbers. He watched them go up and down; "hedging" his bets, the way work had taught him. He was so confident, so in control. He had quickly made friends with the doctors, learned their lingo, found out what the numbers and all the beeping meant, what all the alarms indicated—and he was now in the command center. I had just settled into my chair when a young doctor came up and introduced himself. He proceeded to explain Tayt's situation: how she had had a rough night. How her heart was shunting, her blood gases were remaining low, her sats were not good but were rising. This all made sense to Colin. He had been in the trenches here for twelve hours; listening, figuring out what "shunting", "blood gas", "sats", "meds"—what they all meant. I sat, emotionless, staring at the incubator, which looked more like a tomb to me than anything.

I was drugged out of my mind—not enough to not remember it all, but enough to not feel any of it. Or maybe to feel so much of it that I couldn't handle any more, and shut off. The only time I listened was when the doctor said, "You know, with all the insults that she has endured and the time spent without oxygen, she is going to have some special needs". When we asked exactly what that meant he said, "We just don't know yet". I couldn't help but be overcome with defensiveness. I remember thinking, *How on earth in your world is that relevant?! Shouldn't we make sure she will live long enough to have any needs at all before we talk about special ones?! Aren't there some rules? Like, first you begin with "She is going to live", prior to saying she would have special needs? In what world do people say those sorts of things . . .*

. . . In the world of the NICU, I quickly found out.

There were times when I wished the "special needs" comment was the worst of the insults that were slung. Soon after came the diagnosis of "looks funny" that followed her through her stay. I'm not lying: that was an official diagnosis, that she "looked funny". Not just from a doctor's perspective, either—that comment was from the geneticist. I wasn't aware that "looking funny" was a diagnosis, but, the way that they threw the term around, I am pretty sure that it is in a medical book. Yes, Tayt "looked funny". Her eyes were too small, her fingers were curved, her toes were too long, her head was too small. They started making a physical list of all the traits that made my daughter look funny.

In addition to all the specialists and the tests that were being ordered, there was the team of geneticists. When the authority of the group, Barbara, and her ever-silent assistant (not really mute, I don't think) walked into the NICU, they immediately started with the entire list of "funny" traits that Tayt was exhibiting. Since Tayt had come up so highly linked in my pregnancy blood work with Trisomy 18, they immediately started by telling me that was it. All these traits that she had were associated with that condition. I found *that* funny, going by all the literature I had since read, plus those markers that I had been told time and again she would have, yet didn't (too much space between each toe, curved fingers, little eyes? Nope, nope, nope—none of them here).

Barbara insisted they run her chromosomes. I chimed in that they had run an amniocentesis when I was pregnant. Even if I had ever felt trust in any previous definitive information I had been given in relation to Taytem (which I hadn't), the explanation that followed pulled the chair right out from under me. Apparently, when they do an amniocentesis, it is possible to in fact collect the mother's chromosomes and not those of the fetus. That had not been in my "What to Know About Your Procedure" fact and information sheet! I am quite sure I would have spotted *that* in all those hours I spent waiting in the fetal diagnostic center, stressing over the procedure. As with many tests that they tell you will provide answers, it really only led to more questions. (God alone knows the answers, and He is not administering any of their tests. I have learned the only way to make a medical decision is listen to your heart, listen to your head, and find some answer that you can live with.)

That was all in the first two hours of getting there. My head was pounding and I had hit my mental and physical limit, so I found a bed in a quiet spot in the hospital. I laid down and slept—well, passed out—for twelve hours. When I awoke that day was over and a new one had begun. I found Colin, my poor Colin, still in his chair: still analyzing the numbers, still watching, chewing ice, chewing and smacking his gum loudly, not leaving her side. He never left her side. He sat close, he held her little hand—

He saved her. I believe in my heart that it was his belief in her, his nearness, and his love, that kept her here. From the minute she was born until the minute he would leave this earth, he was her champion. He believed in her in a way that no one else was able to. He loved her, and never felt the need to defend her to anyone; never acknowledged that there was a need.

After a week of showering, changing, and sleeping at the hospital, I realized it was time to go home. I had a life prior to all of this; and, more importantly—most importantly—I had a four-year-old baby at home who was missing his mommy and daddy. So every day, I trudged to the hospital. I would then leave at the crack of dawn and try to get some in-time to spend with Jake. Poor Jake. I was always so afraid for him. I probably ended up ignoring Tayt through some pretty rough patches. I thought at the time she wouldn't miss my absence, but that he would. I would go home at night after two hours of sleep and fight to stay awake just one hour to have a little time for my poor son, who didn't understand what had happened to lead to him losing his parents in an instant.

After about ten days, we believed Tayt was going to make it. If only for a while, the minute-to-minute, hour-to-hour had turned to a stable day-by-day, and she was moved from a one-on-one nurse to a two-on-one setup. She was breathing well with the assistance of the intubation tube and without oxygen, so they decided it was time to remove it and let her breathe on her own. Without the breathing tube, we could start feeding her, take out the NG tube (a tube, inserted through her nose and down to her stomach, which they used to feed her)—and she could come home soon, providing there were no further issues. They took the tube out and immediately we heard that same dreaded noise that had overpowered the delivery room. It sounded like a person trying to breathe through a collapsing straw. It's the sound of a throat buckling under the strain of not having the ability to suck in air. As the stridor got worse, so did her oxygen numbers. Colin and I were whisked away, and when we returned the breathing tube had been shoved back into place—with the operative word being "shoved". After her failed first extubation, and since she "looked funny", we were told she should have a scope to see if her vocal cords were working and/or if there was some anatomical misgivings involved. Once again, we had been brought just to the edge of normalcy, and then yanked away so quickly we hadn't known it was even happening.

She was scheduled for surgery as we waited again to get through this next hurdle. We were told that the specialist who would be doing the bronchoscopy was "the best"—the best in the nation, if not the world. Because this Dr. Holland was such an "important" man, he didn't, following the procedure, have the time to waste on a conference room to update us. He accosted us in the hall and threw out, "She's fine; vocal cords and anatomy were fine; there was just severe edema". I know, right? (It's a fancy-schmancy word for "swelling".) When I asked what was causing it, I was given the *You're wasting my precious time* glance, and told "I don't know".

Here's the important part: we were told her throat looked red, but he didn't think that it warranted antibiotics.

*

Looking back, if you can trace back and identify one moment in your life for a redo, that moment ranks right up there—if not the top one. If I could turn back the clock, I'd insist on antibiotics; to ask him,

"Why not, if not just as a precaution?"

A ten-dollar antibiotic could have potentially cost my daughter seven years of misery, and counting, and no voice.

Yet, back then, it didn't happen like that. Instead he got paged, turned on his heels, and shot his arrogant dust in our bewildered faces.

*

There would be a total of three attempts at extubating poor Tayt. Like clockwork—once, every other day, after another round of steroids—they would try to remove the tube from her throat. They tried every newfangled trick they had. They even put her in a tent with all sorts of steam to moisten her throat. But each time it was to no avail. Within seconds, that loud gasping stridor would sting my ears and involuntarily cause my eyes to water, leaving me crying, unaware, until I felt the sting of salt in my mouth. She remained under five pounds for the next month while every attempt was made to free her from the tube that was sticking out of her mouth. She continued to vomit everything that was being administered through the tube in her nose on a continual basis, which would inevitably end up in her lungs, causing further damage to her little system already so plagued with insult.

Tayt was becoming an ornament at Children's. They moved her into a room with eight babies, where it wasn't unusual to lose one a week. I remember this one nurse, who walked up to one of her babies. She had six vials of different medications to administer at once.

Each was in such perfect balance and in such total dependence on the others that one variation of change could cause a chain of deadly reactions. She did it with such confidence and skill. I will never forget her. Nor will I forget the sadness of someone losing the baby next to us; or coming in to find someone missing and, for self-preservation, assuming they just went home. The NICU is nothing short of a battle zone. You begin to know the people around you. You go from eavesdropping on their situation to finding a way to make a commonality. Misery really does love company.

Taytem had been there long enough at this point to acquire her own nurse. The nurse was the primary caretaker on her case. Her name was Norma. She was heavyset, and about a foot taller and one hundred pounds heavier than me. She sported really bad red short hair—not the real red, but the fake orange "I did it myself" type. If I had to guess, I would say she was probably in her forties; but there are also those people who, because of the harshness that life has handed them, look older than they actually are. That might have been the case with Norma. She had one of those passive-aggressive smiles, and, when she knew someone was watching, she pretended to care a little more about whatever little soul was depending on her for their very life. There was always an undertone in her care that said she felt bothered by their needs, though. For her, nursing did not seem like it was a calling, but possibly the best paycheck she could aspire to. I was there so frequently, and was so concerned about doing everything my way with Tayt's care, that she really just got to sit back and talk my ear off while watching me care for Tayt on my own. I heard all about her son, about her daughter-in-law; their life, their fights . . . all the dirt came out. She was quite the talker. Looking back, however, she was the perfect distraction for me: the perfect thing to throw me off my obsessive behavior, my need to control, my need to fix Tayt.

Then came the day that we were told Tayt's chromosome results were in. We sat in a small room—well, it was more of a closet than a room. I think there were at least fifteen of us in this space, which wasn't really fit for holding more than five. Although I tried to pretend that they weren't there, all these people I didn't know leaned in closer with every word, to hear what my daughter's insides were made from. It was surreal.

"Well, we were really suspicious with Tayt because of the way that she looks and her history." As Barbara the geneticist said this, I rolled my eyes (which, as always, was lost on her). "Normally we only grow out twenty cells, so we did that and they came back normal. But, because of our suspicions about her genetic abnormalities" (again the lost eye roll) "we grew out one hundred, and found one abnormal cell. That is what you would expect to find. But, since she is so abnormal-looking, we didn't feel comfortable that we did a thorough enough job. So . . . we grew out five hundred more, and found one more.

"We don't know what chromosome it is for sure," she continued, "but it LOOKS like an 18, so we believe that she has a Trisomy 18 mosaicism." She proceeded to say that, while it was no longer available for study, Tayt's placenta was hypothesized to contain three 18 chromosomes—although her body didn't. She explained how, when Tayt was being formed, the placenta was made up of the abnormal cells, but that somehow, miraculously, Tayt had been saved. She said that, with time, the good cells in Tayt would continue to multiply, replacing the bad until she was left with only normal cells. She would be normal. We were told that it had only been summarized in theory, because they had never actually seen this in real life. She was one in a million.

Meanwhile, so many failed extubation attempts were starting to be detrimental to her. Her palate was being formed by the tube; her feeding would never happen with the breathing tube in her mouth; it was all snowballing; and nothing would improve until we could get the tube out of her mouth. She was still only four pounds and making no strides on growing or gaining weight. She was so sensitive to the probes, feeding tubes, and trach tubes in her mouth that they would set her into coughing spells, leading even the slightest amount of food that we were able to administer to come up immediately after it went in. If there was edema in her throat causing the trach to remain in, then watching the wrenching and vomiting was enough to know where the majority of it was coming from—yet we were helpless to do anything.

If we didn't at least try to feed her, she would die for sure. I would watch, painstakingly, literally praying, every time 10ccs (which is no more than three droppers full of liquid) would go into her feeding tube. I would then look around, make sure that no one messed with her, make sure that no one disturbed her for minutes, hours on end; only for—*just when* I was quite sure it was finally ingested—her trach to become clogged, which would set off a chain reaction of her coughing, retching, inevitably vomiting, and thereby the whole process would begin again.

We were inoculated, as with everything else in the NICU, into the thought of placing a trach tube for her to breathe until the swelling healed. That way, we could work on the feeding issues and in the meantime worry about her moving around; doing the things that she most certainly needed to start doing; and, above all, coming home. A meeting about what steps needed to be taken for her to be released was scheduled, involving Colin, me, and Dr. Holland and his assistant.

In that meeting, the four of us sat down at the table. The entire time, Holland was shifting, busy, nervous. We were given papers (shoved into our face) to read over, a consent form, and "asked" to sign. We both were bewildered.

"Why do we need to do this? Why does the edema continue?" I asked him. "Isn't there anything else we can do than to put another hole into her?" His answer was a swift "no", him pushing the paper back into our faces, his beeper going off insistently. He wouldn't even take the time to look at us. The assistant looked embarrassed, or scared, but had no further information for us, and simply said,

"So are you ready to sign?"

I don't even think Colin and I glanced at each other. We stood there silently, listening to the sound of our own breathing. We had so many questions, but we swallowed them all. So we did—we signed. We thought we didn't have options. We thought that we had no choice. For the first time ever, I didn't investigate or seek a second opinion. I signed. I just wanted to get her home, and I thought this was the avenue. I made the best decision with the information I had, and after such a long fight, I am embarrassed to say that I was tired and I couldn't fight anymore. I was waving the white flag in exchange for having her home. I always had the thought that, if I could just get her home, I could fix her. I could make it—and her—all better.

The attendant on the NICU floor backed up what Dr. Holland had told us: that we had no other choice but to perform a tracheostomy. To show us how easy and commonplace it was, he took us to see another baby on the floor who had just had the procedure. Things that would have made me sick to my stomach, sights that would have sent me running from a room, were now just that: commonplace. I found nothing shocking anymore. Yet, as I stood over this baby, the calm and pathetic stance that I had grown to have started to fade away, and in an instant I felt like there was a me inside me that just had to run. Looking down at that trach—standing there, feeling the weight of what it represented; the freedom that it took from me, from Tayt, from mine and Colin's once-unencumbered lives—I began to panic inside and feel like I couldn't breathe. I looked to Colin, and he must have seen the terror in my eyes.

Dr. Holland had told me that the trach was temporary. When I had asked "how temporary?" I was told that once the breathing tube was removed, the edema would subside and the trach should only be a couple months' inconvenience at best. One of the respiratory therapists overheard me talking to the nurse about what I was told about the trach duration. I was repeating what the famous Dr. Holland had told me, when she stepped in with a slap of honesty. She told me that, in her experience, once a trach goes in it doesn't come out for years. This same woman had assisted with many of the extubating debacles; had seen the devastation on my face, the tears that ran from my eyes, the lost hope that exuded from my body language as the procedures continued to not work. This nurse had white hair and always wore a white nurse's outfit. While most of the workers on the floor tried to always wear bright colors with stupid Disney characters on their uniforms, she always chose to go with white. She never said much, never seemed to be interested in what was going—or maybe had grown callous from what she saw day in, day out. But here she was, with the first words that I had heard her utter. It was almost as if she just couldn't bear to see me have false hope any longer. She had watched me through this journey, had seen that I could take the truth, and was going to give it to me straight, even if no one else was going to. In the moment I chose to discount her as an angry, bitter old woman who just wanted to be pessimistic—but I now see that she was bucking the system. She was trying to tell me that the doctor was not being honest with me, to save me months—if not years—of angst, of going into appointments expecting the trach to come out.

I wish I had listened to her, picked her brain, given her credit for telling the truth in an atmosphere where that is a career-ender. She hadn't cared; she was deciding to be truthful.

As with all the crap that has been flung at us, we sucked it up, looked past it, and moved on. I went into high gear to get Tayt home. After the damage that was done to her throat; the times I walked in to find her with vomit all over herself; and the times I would see her oxygen had plummeted, only to find her oxygen had come off of her and no one had noticed, I knew it was time to get her out of there.

She would also develop an eye tremor when in hospital, which itself led to us being told that she had probably sustained a brain hemorrhage and therefore had brain damage. When the CAT scan came back normal, they subjected her to an eye exam. Not just any eye exam: they literally took a tool that popped her eye out, so that it then went behind her eyes to make sure they were attached correctly. Again, the results came up aces. It took me doing some research on a new reflux medicine they had her on to tell them that a side effect of overdosing was eye tremors. It was hardly miraculous, therefore, that when they stopped the medicine her eye tremors ceased instantly.

I read Tayt's chart and, as plain as day, it said "Mother is very hard to deal with". Because I told them that the medication they were overdosing her on was causing eye tremors. Because I insisted that edema doesn't just come from nowhere. I was therefore "difficult". I was shut-off by them, and no longer listened to. When I finally felt like we were on our way out the door, I confronted them about it.

Dan Potter was the head attending physician. Dan was an oversized man who had appeared to have the reputation around the ward as the "nice" doctor. He was overbearing, loud, very impressed with himself, and decided that "bucking the system" meant wearing a Hawaiian shirt instead of scrubs and carrying on as if he was on vacation. To some, this came across positively: like he was trying to make himself a man of the people, someone just like us. But I saw it differently.

I think he felt like he had to dumb himself down in order to talk to us. He thought himself so quick-witted, so outrageously smart, that he had to wear ridiculous outfits in order to fit in among "us folk". He was condescending, and rude, with a big old mustache and a Texan accent that boomed when he talked. He had this stupid phrase (again, which I can imagine him practicing in the mirror, ensuring it came off as being dumbed-down enough)—that the kids in the NICU were "Dan's kids"; insisting he treated them all as if they were his own.

Anyhow, I finally confronted him as he was sitting in his office. He looked over to me, standing in the doorway, and invited me to have a seat. I thought carefully about my choice of words. After being in the ward as long as I had, I discovered that anything past niceties makes you someone who is unreasonable. Questioning an opinion, inquiring more, came across as being obstinate, and that was threatening to the entire atmosphere. I started speaking very calmly, careful not to show the emotion that I felt and the protective mother's bear claws that are so instantaneous and lasting. When you have as many people in one space thinking you are a raving lunatic, all feeling like you clearly have a screw loose, well, then you don't often tend to question others. And so, for someone like me—who is so incredibly sensitive and concerned about what people think of me—this urge was new. Not caring about how I would come across, instead caring more about defending someone else, had now became my new normal.

In that tiny office, I found my voice and used it. I began in the most polite and respectful way to tell Dan that I was offended by the way that he treated me with such flippant comebacks. I told him that I understood that it is a hospital setting where you have to say what things are, but that as the parent of a child, speaking about a child's appearance with such lack of empathy, or awareness that we have feelings, should be rethought. I continued to tell him that if they were "Dan's kids", as he so often claimed, then Dan should consider how he would like someone calling his kid the many hurtful and dismissive things that he had said about my daughter during rounds, in meetings, and while with associates. I needed him to know that his comments had dehumanized Tayt, and with his words he made it possible to make decisions and calls that were not coming from a place of professionalism; and they robbed Tayt of the compassion that she deserved. When I left his office, I had very little confidence that my words made an impact, but he had impacted me and my experience and so I felt like it had needed to be said, if only for my own peace of mind.

I had known immediately after the trach was placed that it was time to get her home. But with the trach came a whole host of other problems. These were issues that we had not been forewarned of prior to its placement, when the doctors had been so insistent that the trach was the sole solution to her throat problem.

First, there was the practical issue that she could not come home until Colin and I could maintain it.

To make matters worse, with the trach also came a gut-wrenching "cough". Although she had exhibited this prior to its placement, the insertion of the trach greatly exacerbated it. She would cough, every seven to ten minutes, so violently that she would vomit.

Moreover, although we had at some point gotten her up to a whopping five pounds with the introduction of the trach and the placement of her G-tube (a gastrostomy tube that extended to her stomach so that food could be fed to her without her having to eat), she now needed to be watched around the clock. She had to be watched because she had to be fed constantly. We literally had to take an extension tube and push food directly into her stomach, because she was down to four pounds by the age of ten weeks. The gastrostomy tube did nothing to keep the food in, so it was a cycle—us pumping food in; her vomiting it out, almost instantaneously. The doctors added a "venting" bag onto the gastrostomy bag, so that whatever she ate and then threw up would be pushed back up the tube and sit until it could go back in. She would regurgitate food all day. The same 60ccs (about two ounces) of food would be pushed through the G-tube at the beginning of every morning and then be pushed back out and in again for about twelve hours. We had just about every specialty consultation that you can think of: pulmonologist, gastroenterologist, anesthesiologist, neurologist, ophthalmologist, geneticist—the list was vast. Finally, an endocrinologist consult was requested; him being called for because of her inability to gain weight, and because she was growing very slowly.

We knew she didn't have any of the genetic issues that would be causing the failure to gain weight, so we hoped maybe the endocrinologist might try to figure out if she had a metabolic problem. He had ordered some tests, which had all come back fine. When he came into her room, he peered into her little crib, looked at her, pulled up her cover, then turned her over a couple of times. Both Colin and I were waiting, watching, hoping that the wizard was going to speak. After looking very thoughtful—like he was really giving it true consideration—he looked over at us and said, "She is going to be small". I kid you not, that was exactly what he said. "She is going to be small."

Being the smart ass that I am, I asked him: "Are we talking Barbie-doll size? Do I need to get her a Barbie Jeep to take to school?"

This he found completely and utterly insulting, as if I was making light of his professional opinion.

"I can't tell you exactly how small," he responded. "All I know is that she is growing slowly and probably will continue to. There is nothing in her blood work that I can see."

With that, he headed out of the room. Colin and I stood silent for a minute, looking at one another like *What just happened here?* before we then both erupted into laughter. Though the not-so-funny part of the story is the Ben for $350 that came to our home a month later for that professional opinion.

At this point, the medical bills were beginning to mount, babysitting costs were starting to rack up, and Colin—who wanted to help me out and not leave Tayt's side—nevertheless had to return to work or else we wouldn't be able to keep the house. And so he returned to work, while I went back to trying to get Tayt home. She couldn't come home without nursing care, but our insurance company was saying that she didn't need nursing. This is the glitch that no one knows about until they have a child with a major medical issue. I finally contacted an agency run through the University of Illinois to help get her home. It was a state-run agency that would pay her nursing costs. We had been working with a social worker (who must have been married to the endocrinologist, because she was about as helpful), who had never even suggested it. By the time I found it, we were already two weeks past the G-tube placement surgery, and there was an eight-to-ten-week wait to get her covered and get her home.

Chapter Nine

Sometimes I say that I am "angry", but I've begun to see that frustration is so much worse. With anger, there is someone to blame. There is something to fight against—if not physically, then at a minimum emotionally—and that gets you somewhere, because you get to displace it. But where does frustration go?

That's the thing: there is no way to push frustration off. You are in a cycle that isn't changeable or fixable—it is just more of the same. The definition of insanity is doing the same thing and expecting a different result. What is frustration then, if it's not doing the same thing, never expecting it to change or get better, but being trapped by it anyway? If so, frustration is quickly becoming my life.

*

Although I had applied for nursing through the state and this most assuredly would be approved, they were dragging their heels over it. I was convinced at the time that we didn't have time; that she didn't have that kind of time. I therefore manned the wagons and started circling. I threatened BCBS that I would sue. They laughed. I'm sure that their lawyers had ironclad writing in our policy outline. I threatened to go to the media, and again they scoffed. So that's what I did. I wrote Oprah, and I called NBC, ABC, Fox, and CBS, trying to get our story heard. I got a call back from CBS, seemingly showing some interest, only to be yelled at by the famous newsmaker on the phone. "You are going after them because they are paying for your hospitalization?" they said. "Lady, consider yourself lucky." Then *click*. Finally, NBC returned my message. I got word that they were going to come by and tape our story.

Come the filming day, I hadn't gotten dressed up, put on makeup, even brushed my hair in God knows how long, but I really didn't care about the prospect of being seen on the ten o'clock news all over Chicago. I had but one goal in getting on the news: to shame the insurance company, to whom I paid my premium, that would not pay to bring my baby home.

The crew came to the house. It was just the reporter and a cameraman. They put the camera literally up to our faces. They sat Colin and I in a tiny chair each. You don't realize, watching people on television, how close that camera comes—far past your personal-space boundary. First we told our story, and then they had Jake run around hitting balls in the backyard. I remember thinking, *Really, my daughter is dying in the hospital and I am begging you to help me get her home . . . and you are making me take my four-year-old outside and having him run around the backyard, as if that relates at all to the fact that the insurance company won't pay their share? What is this world all about?* It was so warped, but I played their game. We all learn to play the game, don't we? That is why some people get ahead in life and some don't—they learn to play the game, or to rise above it. Those who do neither, well, they survive, but not very successfully.

As I say, several weeks before she was released, we had decided that, to help get Tayt home, a gastronomy tube (G-tube) would be a good option. The doctors would do a surgical procedure to move her stomach to the surface of her body and insert a G-tube, which would be like a portal straight to her stomach. We were told the surgery would be easy, but as for the recovery . . . well, not so much fun. If we didn't agree to placing the G-tube, we would have to continue feeding her with a nasogastric tube (NG-tube), which was inserted into her nose and down her esophagus hundreds of times a day and was doing nothing to save her throat from further damage, and so again we signed her life away—literally. Every time she would cough the NG-tube would come out of her nose and catapult itself onto her shirt. This action would lead whatever nurse was around to grab her by the face, look her in the eye, and push that tube right back into her nose. Not just into her nose, mind you, but the tube literally had to be inserted deeply into her nasal cavity to reach her stomach. Tayt would be flailing the whole time, her eyes wide and fixed on the wall, and every time there would be one minuscule tear in her eye. I think the most heart-wrenching moment was when she eventually stopped flailing and stopped crying. It was like they had broken her spirit. I understood that because I was near to breaking myself. I was barely holding on, and to see her lose her hope, her belief in a life outside of this, made me think maybe there wasn't one.

Come this point I had grown completely skeptical of the hospital's ability to take care of Tayt. I would have nightmares that they killed her. That they gave her the wrong medicine. That they let her oxygen slide, and I would come in to find her eyes not looking at me anymore. That was the thing—as time went on, Tayt was overcoming what they told us she would be. In spite of all the insult her body endured, she did everything on time. She followed us and the nurses around the room. Nothing got past those little watchful eyes. She saw and understood everything. And I was so *afraid* of losing that. I honestly felt that if they did something by mistake, they would cover it up; they would lie; they would say she never had the ability from the get-go and go back to their global "something wrong" diagnosis to blame it on. I was becoming increasingly paranoid. I was panicked to just get her home. I sat there, hours a day, for months. What I witnessed happen to other babies never got reported, and I am sure was never told to the parents who couldn't be there twenty-four-seven. But mistakes happened, and were quickly swept under the rug.

The date came for the placement of Tayt's G-tube, and Colin and I were there early. Although it was what we were told was the final step to being able to get her home, it was one that I was not entirely sold on. They wheeled her out in her incubator and her eyes were filled with fear. As they took her down the corridor, she was watching Colin and me following behind her. She was in a position that looked unnatural: constantly searching for us, never letting us out of her sight until they took her in. We were told it would be a forty-five-minute procedure, and, as we had now become accustomed to, we settled into the tiny, humid, smelly waiting room. The odor of perspiration, fear, and angst hung in the air. I watched the clock intently. Thirty minutes went by . . . no word. One hour . . . I began shifting in my chair, arms crossed. I felt Colin getting anxious, but we both remained patient. Sometimes things just took longer. Then another hour. And then sheer dread set in. We were both panicked and paralyzed. After this long journey, was it really going to end here? With a decision that we elected to go for? Was this where it would end after two months of fighting to get her home? We should have gone up to the desk to confirm what was happening, but we were both too afraid to ask.

After three hours had passed, I was in tears—assuming the worst had happened. One of the assistants to the general surgeon came over to sit down. He had such an odd look on his face. I thought, *Here we go, they are breaking the new kid in, getting him to administer the bad news.* In the most nonchalant, flippant tone, he said, "Why are you guys still down here? Tayt was moved upstairs over two hours ago. Didn't anyone tell you?" I could feel Colin and me collectively hit the ceiling of what our bodies could contain. Just like that, our boiling point had been reached. All I remember is security threatening to eject us, Colin demanding to see the surgeon directly, and then the four of us being put in an empty room to discuss what had happened. Colin had let eight weeks of pent-up anger, angst, frustration, terror—all of it—explode over this surgeon. He had previously maintained his cool whenever I was screaming at doctors, telling them where they could go, what I thought of them. Colin had stood behind me to hold me up. He was always stood in my cheering section: always on my side, but never stealing my thunder, never stifling my need to let it all out. But this was his turn. He had finally had enough. This was the last straw.

He towered over this surgeon, whose pager was going off countless times yet who didn't have the guts to look at it. Colin got right up in his face: spit flying from his mouth, his eyes wide with rage. He was talking about how this man thought he was so important, with his nice shoes, and his nice suit, but he wasn't anything special. His ability to cut someone up, that was nothing special. How the way he had let us sit there, thinking that Tayt was dead—the way that he had just gone about his business—made him an awful human being: a callous and awful human being. I stood silent. I agreed with it all. I hope Colin felt me standing behind him, holding him up.

Retelling that story doesn't do it justice. I have the entire vision in my head: this chief of surgery puffing out his chest, trying to exert his superiority; Colin taking him down like on an episode of *SmackDown*. Again, the surgeon threatened to call security. How dare we talk to the almighty that way! We had broken code, and now we were *both* "very difficult". We would tell that story so many times over the years. I always recounted it with a smile, because I pictured it as the day Colin "stooped to my level", and I knew it was as cathartic for him as it was me.

The problem was that if we took Tayt home before she was approved by the state for aid, I would be admitting that I didn't need help. I would have to sign papers to say I was declining assistance, and you can't ever go back from that. Therefore I had to wait, and I had to badger. I was young and obstinate and completely willing to sign the papers to take her home, to take over her care . . . but thank goodness I was mature enough by this point to know that to do that would be to jeopardize her safety. So, after waiting so long, I finally got the call that the nursing had been approved, and we were on our way to getting her home. The next hurdle was finding the nursing. There was a nursing shortage, which meant that the agencies were staffing insurance cases first. There were no nurses left to staff state cases. We finally found one who would take us, but I had to guarantee to personally pay the $5-per-hour difference between what the state and private insurance reimburses. At the time Colin was making a good living, but twenty-four hours of $5/hr was more money than we could possibly afford. But I felt I didn't have any other choice. I signed the discharge papers, and we only had about half of the necessary staffing at home, but it was enough to get her home where she belonged.

Two days before she was scheduled to come home, the NBC story ran on the news. In our interview, they had called me prior to airing to find out whether there were any additions to the story. I had told them that she was coming home, and I told them all about the guarantee that I gave to the nursing agency to pay the difference. They added that information to the end of the commentary on the news story. The significance of this was that—unbeknownst to me, although I can't imagine to the agency—it was illegal. Technically it was "insurance fraud", and now I could be prosecuted. Luckily, the papers were torn up. The nursing company, to save face, insisted that they had "no idea", and the nurse began taking the monies from the state case without the additional out-of-pocket portion from us.

Chapter Ten

I've heard it said that writers aren't created, they are a product of their experiences—both the good and the heartbreaking—but that isn't entirely true. Some of us naturally see a situation unfold within a fleeting second, and imagine various versions of the ending, with these always larger-than-life, written descriptively, felt immensely. Empathy is a necessity for humans to survive, there is no doubt about that. But there are some of us who have gotten bigger doses of it. Feeling for everyone is both a blessing and a curse. I would imagine that not being an empathetic being is like a meal without seasoning. Is that a good thing, or bad? Colin and I are cut from the same extra-empathetic cloth, which, when combined, at times makes it even harder.

Everyone keeps responding to our blog, telling us that our story is a beautiful love story. I never thought of us in that light. We've never been the holding hands, lovey-dovey kind of couple, but I am starting to realize how connected our souls are and always have been. We are the type of couple where if I had found myself thinking *We should have tacos for dinner* . . . Colin would then come home with Taco Bell. We share a common wavelength. We have the same thoughts, the same feelings. There have also been times during his illness when I myself have been nauseated, or have a headache beyond belief. I have been told they are sympathy pains, yet I don't believe that. I believe that our souls have been so joined together that we feel for each other, truly feel what the other is feeling. If there were ever two people who are meant to be together it would be us. While driving with my mother the other day, I recounted how so many years back I ran into Colin in the bar downtown—where our lives together really started. After all of the years being separated throughout high school and college, meeting up with him felt like "coming home". I had, over the following six months, done all that I could to avoid a relationship with him that was anything more than friendship, though I couldn't ever really say why. Examining my feelings in retrospect, I believe that there was so much fear in feeling that connected to someone, or perhaps even relying on them, that kept me at arm's length. Maybe I sensed the pain of the journey that we would have together. Maybe, all those years ago, I knew what we would have to endure, but didn't know why, and didn't know whether I was up for the challenge. Yet, somewhere along the line, I realized that, without him, without him as my partner, life wouldn't be worth living. I chose him knowing the course we would have to go down. How could I exist without him now?

*

I went home to get the "nursery" ready. I took a trip to Pottery Barn Kids and loaded up on the most feminine, expensive, top-of-the-line nursery décor I could find to decorate her room to the hilt. I stayed up all night, putting Jake's old crib together. When Colin tried to interrupt me—asking why I was so frantic, getting the room ready when I wasn't sure when she was coming home—I exploded. Two months of rage burst from me, all wrapped into some silly argument, which left Colin looking at me like I was crazy.

The months of angst and turmoil, watching the daughter I gave birth to being tortured. There was a tube in every part of her, to do all of the things she should have been able to do on her own. Yet here we sat, without a single reason as to *why*. There was no reason she had been sick, or why her throat was swollen. Why was all of this happening to her? I had to get her home. She needed to be home with us, so that I could start over. In my head if, I could just get her home, I could fix her. I believed it, I knew it. I could save her.

So it was true: Tayt was going to finally come home. The nursing agency showed up at our house the Friday before we brought her back. The medical supply people came over with everything she would need. I'd had the entire room decorated ready for my daughter 's arrival. I was still holding onto the fantasy that everything was going to be fine. I still had dreams that, in two years, I wouldn't even remember what came before. But when they pulled the van up, they quickly turned my fairy-tale-princess room into an extension of the NICU. The bedding had to be moved for tubes. The curtains had to be moved for the feeding pump; the dresser for the oxygen tank. The latter looked like a missile in the corner of her room. The machines were aligned with her bed: not just the feeding pump, but the humidifier, the O2 SAT machine. Her room was no longer the perfect nursery room, but the perfect remote hospital room. Still, she was coming home.

I remember the medical supply people painstakingly going over what I had to do: how I would hook everything up, what level everything had to be at, what I had to watch for, what I had to change once a day, once a week, once a month. I sat, pretending to listen, but was not hearing a word of it. I was overwhelmed, and I didn't even know it. After they left all the new mess behind, I cried that night as I looked around the room. I had wanted her home so badly, but I had so much guilt. Colin and I had had a conversation two weeks after she was born. We were sitting at a bar down the street from the hospital: the same bar we used to go to enjoy ourselves many times; being overserved, laughing, not a care in the world. And here we now were—well, we could scratch that bar off our list of happy places. I looked at Colin with tears streaming down my face. I said that it felt like Tayt had just had plastic surgery. Yes, she was alive, but it would take a while to unravel the bandages in order to see what we had. Yes, we had saved her, but at what cost? Should we really have done that? Morally, should we save babies at any cost? What would our lives become?

The next day was finally "pick up day", and we were at last going to take her home. I was a nervous wreck. Her medical issues all seemed so doable—until they had brought all the same materials to our home, at which point it had all looked so overwhelming.

*

Our calling the television news seemed like it had been a waste of time, only years later I met up with a woman who lived close to me. My friend had introduced us, thinking that we could help each other out. She had a boy with a trach: a young boy who lived very close to us. The boy was released within six months from when Tayt had come home from the hospital. When I asked her if she had a hard time getting her son nursing, she said to me "Oh we got lucky, there was some family who was on the news about Blue Cross Blue Shield not paying for their daughter's trach. Afterward, the insurance company had to reverse their decision about our son and pay after it aired". I'd like to believe that was the universe evening out.

*

The nursing was set up. We were supposed to have sixteen hours a day, but, because of the nursing shortage, and since we were state and not private insurance funded, our case was not high on the priority list. Our required sixteen hours a day (one hundred and twelve hours a week) were turned into just sixteen hours a week. We had one day nurse for three days a week, who would work from nine a.m. till three p.m.; and then one night nurse, who would work Monday through Thursday from eleven p.m. to six a.m.—a total of forty-six hours' help per week, of which only sixteen were now to be covered by the state. That also left the other four daytimes just to me, and the three leftover nights to me as well. It sounded doable... until I realized that I wouldn't be able to sleep. There was no time left for sleep! By this point Colin had returned to work and so was unable to stay up all night long, and nor was he available during the day.

To watch Tayt was not like watching another child. I literally had to stand over her, watch her every breath, and feed her around the clock, but at the same time watch that she didn't vomit it up, which she did at least ten times a day. If the vomiting started, I had to make sure she wasn't aspirating it. In the hospital they talked about it all the time, but I had no idea that was really lingo for causing pneumonia. Aspirating it would mean her ending up in the hospital for a three-week stint, or dying. So I had to stand over her, keeping watch. And then there was my poor son Jake. At the age of four, he just wanted my attention; he just wanted to play. He didn't understand why I couldn't leave her side; he just wanted some of my time.

Wayne, the nurse who was first assigned to cover days, showed up every morning that he worked with a bad ego and some gym shorts that were clearly way, way too short. There was rumor from the other nurses who worked with us that he had had some "mail-order" bride from Russia who ran off on him, but we couldn't ever confirm it. He would sit in that little room with Tayt, and while he was there I would try to go out and get Jake out of the house. But every time I would come home, he was glued to the television; he wouldn't even acknowledge us coming in the door. I would look into the crib to find that Tayt had vomited all over herself and he hadn't noticed—probably hadn't even looked. If I truly want to be honest with myself, I knew he was not taking care of Tayt. I knew she was not safe; I wouldn't have let him watch Jake, even. But I needed the time away. I needed the time with Jake. I couldn't lose him in an attempt to save Tayt.

That was the summer of 2001, and September 11th. Jake had started back at preschool, and I went into Tayt's room to find Wayne watching the planes hit the towers a thousand times. He was attached to that television. He didn't move, he didn't flinch, he didn't check on Tayt, or feed her, or change her. He sat in front of the television until I finally said, "That's enough. You are going to have to leave now". Completely stunned, he gathered his things and stormed out.

Now we had to try to find a new nurse, and would spend the next two months going through several more of them. They would send temporary replacements for Wayne. Some would come once, some twice, but none of them ever stayed. Tayt was still throwing up and going to the hospital frequently. Every trip involved her oxygen, her suction machine, and pitying glances. We had crazy nurse after scary nurse. Some often didn't show at all, and others I was afraid to leave her alone with.

In the fall of her homecoming, Tayt had developed a crick in her arm: something I had originally noticed shortly after she came home. I noticed one day, as I sat staring at her, that she never moved her right arm at all. At the time Tayt was only four months, but when she lay on her back and looked up at toys, she only reached with her left arm. It was like she didn't even know she had a right arm. Of course, I quickly went to work on trying to diagnose this new finding. I was instantly sure that someone had broken her arm at Children's and had said nothing. I took her to our pediatrician, along with all the equipment that involved: oxygen machine, suction machine, trach cover—it was like touring a small circus. The cue him staring, the look of confusion as to what was wrong with Tayt, the pity—only to have him tell me that she was fine. He told me I was overreacting. That, if there was something there, we would not know until she was much older and had more developed skills. In his estimation, there was nothing we could do, plus it was probably nothing. Even if it wasn't, it was something that we had to wait out and something that we could do nothing about. But I didn't agree.

Early Intervention, a program to help kids with setbacks, had allowed me to request a physical therapy consult. I took her to the physical therapist just as fall was turning to winter. Looking back on it, it was really a risky trip, considering her respiratory weakness. But there I met Joe: a therapist trained in Chile, and a woman who was one of a handful of people in Tayt's life who I truly believe saved her from a lifetime of disability. The first physical therapist that I saw told me she was too young for me to worry about her arm, there was nothing really that could be done. Joe believed in the brain connection of the young. I took Tayt for x-rays, and when no break was detected we quickly determined that this was the beginning stages of hemiparesis (cerebral palsy on one side). She had all the classic symptoms, and we both believed that if we could retrain her brain and bridge whatever damage had been done, then her outcome would be so much better. Just as her right arm had stopped being used, so too did the right leg. I had no training besides determination, but I began to tie down her left arm. I physically took string and I tied down her left arm to her side with nylons to force her brain to use the right. I had one nurse refuse to work with me. She told me that I was being abusive. But I didn't care; I persisted. Slowly but surely, Tayt began using that right arm.

Soon she had gone from not using her right arm at all, to using both arms the same amount. Over time, I missed several appointments for Tayt—we were in and out of the hospital all the time, so I felt alright about missing some of her exams, rechecks, and checkups—but I never missed her therapy sessions. Joe would tell me to massage her right foot, to help her motions become more fluid, as they naturally should, but yet didn't for Tayt. When she sat up, the left side was so much weaker and the movements so much more immature. I spent day and night massaging, pushing, tying. I was obsessed. I couldn't control much with Tayt. I couldn't control her getting sick, her inability to eat, her poor weight gain, her vomiting; but this was something I could control. This was something I knew something about, something that I felt I could change, so I kept at it. I massaged night after night until her clenched hand opened up and her immature movements became fluid.

Along with her physical therapy, she had speech therapy. That didn't go so well. She worked with the same woman who would come round, put something into Tayt's mouth, gag her, Tayt would throw up, and then the therapist would start over. Since all Tayt really did was throw up, it wasn't anything alarming, but I didn't see the point in it. The therapist would come for an hour, gag her three times, and tell me I needed to "desensitize her upper palate" (which really translated into "gag her on your own three times, three times a day"). I guess the assumption was that, if we desensitized the oral area enough, Tayt would eventually stop gagging. Unfortunately, it never worked. She never stopped gagging, even to this day.

When Tayt was about eleven months old, she was officially labeled as "failure to thrive" (which really means "we don't know and we don't care", and basically "it's no longer our problem or fault"). She still had the trach, and I would take her in month after month to the do the scans of her throat, where I would cry and plead with Dr. Holland to tell me why she kept vomiting. Finally, after meeting with the gastroenterologist, we decided to put in a J-tube. She already had a G-tube (where the tube was flush up to the stomach exterior), but the

J-tube would be put in, its position checked via x-ray, and it would then inject food straight into the large intestine, so that she couldn't throw it up. It seemed like the perfect solution: now, whatever she was fed would bypass her stomach. We would start feeding her food that was already broken down, and place it immediately into the large intestine. So, they placed the tube and we went home.

Back at home following the J-tube's insertion, Tayt was miserable. Even though she had been through so much, she was normally a delightful ham. With the exception of what her medical condition demanded from us, she wanted for nothing. She really never cried, nor required our attention; in fact, she almost wanted to be on her own. But she was always happy, and always entertaining. Well, within two hours of the J-tube's being placed, she looked miserable and in pain. She spent the next couple of hours vomiting. Of course, this was no different from before—yet it *was* supposed to be different now. The placement of the tube was supposed to stop the vomiting. Not only did it not, but the vomiting appeared more painful, became more frequent; and, although it contained no food, it went from being dry heaves to a green-colored substance.

After eighteen hours of watching her throw up bile, I returned to Children's to be told I hadn't given the J-tube enough time to work. They convinced me to give it just a little while longer, and in the meantime they hospitalized her. I sat in the hospital while we were told, over and over again, "Sometimes it just takes some time to work". After five days, I brought her back home—no better, still throwing up—while I was told to *just wait*, just wait; to stop being so paranoid, crazy, and difficult—and if I would just let them do their job, she would be fine.

Within ten hours of being home, she was lifeless and unresponsive. I took her back to the emergency room once again. I told them I wanted the tube removed. When they refused, I insisted that I was leaving. (There is a hidden fact in our hospitals—that you can leave whenever you want. You are not a prisoner. When you are in the hospital you can leave anytime you want.) So that is what I did. I finally said to them that I didn't trust them to touch her again, and I was out of there.

The next morning, I called Colin at work and said, "I am leaving; I am taking Taytem to Mayo Clinic". We knew that neither the advice we were getting at Children's Hospital nor the specialists that we were seeing were helping. They weren't doing her any good. Colin asked me if I had an appointment, as we had been trying to make an appointment there. It is not easy to get in to Mayo. I said I didn't, but I was going to the emergency room and they had to take us. Colin rushed home, and at five on a Friday we hopped into the car and drove from Chicago to Minnesota, speeding all the way in a beat-up, crappy Nissan that I was afraid would not make the five-hour trip. Tayt was in the backseat, with Colin riding alongside her. She had just enough energy to lift her gaze to look at him. She needed to keep looking to see it in his eyes: to see his belief that she was going to make it, that she was going to live. I did the same: looking into the rearview mirror and searching out his gaze, the same reassurance that she was going to survive.

Colin had a way, when he looked to me, of letting me know that everything was going to be okay, that all was not lost. Tayt's story was not going to end here, in a beat-up shitty Nissan Sentra passed down from my mother, breaking down in the middle of the highway. It would all be alright.

*

He looks to me in these final months, the way that I did to him in the rearview mirror of that car, and in so many other times of crisis. His gaze fixed upon me, begging me, begging for me to save him, to tell him everything is going to be alright, that his story is not going to end. But I can't return the favor, and it leaves me with a heavy heart.

Chapter 11

Using the term "malpractice" will get you kicked out of a hospital, much like yelling "bomb!" will on a plane. Malpractice doesn't necessarily mean that you are going to sue, or there is going to be litigation: sometimes it just means that things go wrong. I can imagine that things go wrong all of the time. In all of our lives, we make mistakes at work—albeit, for most of us, those mistakes don't change the course of someone's life or affect their ability to function.

Years later, I can honestly say that I have never had so many mishaps happen to one person as I have seen with Tayt. Sometimes I wonder whether she is the luckiest or the unluckiest person—or the unluckiest of the luckiest people—in the universe. Nothing is never "normal" or fair for her. When I come home with fast food for everyone, Tayt's is always the order that is missing. If something can go wrong, it will. But in many ways, those "mistakes" have also been the things that have allowed her to defy the odds in positive ways. Every time there is a big Lotto pot, I take her to the store and give her a ticket to fill out. Just once, she has to hit it big, right? Not yet, but we keep playing.

JULIE BARTH

*

We entered the Mayo emergency room and begged yet another group of doctors to please save her life. By the time we arrived there Tayt was unresponsive, listless, literally dying. She had had nothing to eat that had stayed in her body and not excreted through bile or urine in almost two weeks. Within two hours of our arrival at the Mayo Clinic, the doctors removed the J-tube. They told us that Children's had placed an adult-sized tube into our seven-pound baby girl. By this time, she was back down to five pounds and eight ounces. She had lost the weight we'd so painstakingly put on over the past couple of months. The nurse who came in to see Tayt in the wee hours of the evening told us that, if we had not gotten her there when we did, she would have died within the next twelve hours. Then one of the nurses went out on a limb to tell us that what the other hospital did had almost killed Tayt. She told us that they had made a HUGE mistake; and she took the tube, put it into an envelope, told us that she would not help us directly because it was a strict no-no, but that the tube was our proof of what they had done. She should have had an infant-size 16cc, and they put an adult 16cc in. That's a range from a newborn to a two-hundred-pound-man-size tube. I still have the tube. I figure I will keep it for Tayt for when she is of age if she wants to pursue it.

We stayed at the Mayo Clinic for over two weeks that first time. After four days we had Colin's stepfather drive Jake to come meet us. Mayo is surrounded by many things to do—it is a hospital built around the idea that it is housing people who don't live there—so we were able to get a room near a waterpark. It was almost like a mini vacation for all of us, as weird as that sounds. Tayt finally had the round-the-clock nursing she needed. We felt safe. As one of us stayed with her, the other spent undivided time with Jake. He even got to ride in a helicopter, which he still remembers.

This hospital was different. There was no drilling or construction going on. There was an incredible system in place for transport, tests, and scheduling. You were never there any longer than you needed to be, nor did you have to wait for hours on end. Here, we would never have been left in a surgery waiting room without being contacted. Over those sixteen days, we saw a whole new team of the same set of specialists. They were more concerned about what had happened since she was born. We did also do another genetic workup: seeing more geneticists, going through syndrome registries—the whole nine yards—and were still unable to find one single thing that was not related to the treatment (or lack thereof). The ENT who examined her throat on the third day confirmed my worst fears. All those months ago, when Tayt first had the scope and Dr. Holland told us there was nothing wrong with her vocal cords, he had not been telling the truth. We knew that the worst that could happen was if her vocal cords were not working. We were shattered to find out that, in fact, through scarring or through infection, her vocal cords had ceased to function. We finally found out that Tayt's trach was not coming out any time soon. She would have the trach for a very long time—maybe forever.

After the initial relief of finally being told the truth, the devastation and anger intensified and burned in my soul. The ENT continued to tell us that the only way for Taytem to live without the trach was to have surgery—major reconstructive surgery, which would span two or three procedures. She explained to us that Taytem had what is termed "vocal cord fixation". Her vocal cords could vibrate, so she would be able to talk without the trach, but its being fixated meant that she couldn't breathe without it. She continued by telling us that they did have a new procedure, whereby they would tack back one of the vocal cords. This would not jeopardize Tayt's ability to talk, and would allow her to breathe. The ENT added that she believed that the reason Tayt threw up as much as she did was because somewhere along the way Tayt had sustained brain damage, which caused her to not be able to swallow correctly. We would need a "swallow study" to verify this. She also added that she had seen someone who looked like Tayt, and who had the same features; she couldn't remember who or where, but she insisted she had seen someone like Taytem.

We walked out of that room shellshocked. All that we had known and had been told for the past year were lies. As he always was, Colin was able to make it okay for me. He assured me that we would be able to fix this. He promised me that there would be a time when she would live without a trach. I knew that, unlike most people, he wasn't just saying it; he believed it. In his heart, he always believed in Tayt like no one else has or ever could.

Chapter 12

As I visit Colin at his parents' house, I realize I have gotten to the point whereby I don't even pick up the phone anymore; where I can't stand to talk about it anymore, so quickly and so easily does the devastation well up and then overflow. I feel like I am suffocating. There was a time right after he started treatment that Colin would tell people that I "saved his life". But here I sit, watching him die.

I got here and we decided to change his clothes.

"I don't care who sees me anymore," he said.

"Who's looking at you Colin?" I replied, sure that he was hallucinating.

"No, I just don't care about being naked anymore."

"Nothing I haven't seen before," I replied, before quickly heating up some wash up cloths in the microwave and returning to start changing his clothes.

He is literally skin and bones. He looks thin with clothes on, but it's the bones protruding through the skin when the clothes are gone that I can't believe. I stand looking at him, waiting to hear what I could do next.

"So, that's it? We aren't going to do anymore blood work?" he says.

"For what? Why do you want more blood work?"

"So they're just going to let me die then, they are just letting me…" He trails off, making the chop of the neck sign with his hand.

"No, Colin, if you want them to run your blood work, all you have to do is ask."

"I am tired, can you move my leg up?"

So I do, and off to sleep he goes.

I have been beating myself up, for giving up on trying to save Colin at all costs, as I sit here and realize how incredibly much he fights, how much more he has to fight. Had I known—had I known how much he has left in him—we would not be here. I was talking to the one friend who I can continue to talk to.

"I let him down Laura. Had I known he had so much more fight, I should have investigated, I should have gotten him into another trial, I should have fought harder for him than I did instead of throwing in the towel and watching him whittle away."

"But you did everything," she assures me instantly. "He was so sick. I know you are forgetting, but he was so sick. Any further treatment would have robbed you of the time you have had, and the time you have left now."

"Evidently not," I shoot back. "Now I have to just watch and let him die in front of me. That is something I will have to live with. All of those trips with Taytem to different hospitals. He believed in her, we did. Why didn't I give him the same benefit of the doubt?"

"Because you know saving him is not possible. You know he has already given all that he had and it was his time."

*

We came out of the meeting with Thomas, the young ENT doctor at Mayo. Although I believed most of it because it made sense, I was really hung up on her "brain damage" swallow theory. I just couldn't see how Tayt was able to keep up with all of her milestones on time, yet had sustained enough brain damage to not even be able to swallow.

Following the meeting they came for Tayt, took her off to the exam room, put a camera down her throat, and then proceeded to put blue dye into her mouth to see where it went. It was a disaster. She began vomiting and fighting. Although she was a tiny little thing, she was definitely strong, and you really saw it when she was held down. And so the spontaneous and disastrous swallow study came up empty. It was neither a confirmation nor a denial, and had effectively been an exercise in "let's just see what we have here". Thomas decided maybe this approach hadn't the best route to take after all, and that it should in fact be planned and more controlled. Another test was therefore scheduled.

A couple of days later, we could see that Tayt was coming around. The child-sized J-tube had since been placed correctly, and she was finally returning to life. She was sitting up, laughing, joking with nurses. She would make faces and laugh and play jokes. She needed no language—she still had no voice—but we knew exactly what she was saying. She was engaging, fun, and so darn cute.

After being there for a couple of days we finally—for the first time—saw her eat. I came in from the hotel to see Colin at Tayt's beside. He had a bowl of Cheerios and applesauce in his hand, and was spoon-feeding it to Tayt. They both looked up at me like it was nothing new and she had done it for a lifetime. Colin informed me that they had just gotten back from the second swallow study. In my absence—which was probably a good thing—they had taken Taytem to a room, and in an unobtrusive way had provided her applesauce and Cheerios and asked her to eat them. With Colin at her side, she had done it: she had eaten and she had swallowed.

"Did she vomit a lot?" I asked Colin.

"Not at all," he said, beaming. "They were definitely wrong about the brain damage theory."

The findings of the second swallow test were pretty easy. We were told that, basically, her vocal cords were fixated—as had been previously stated—but that, with time and with the right surgeries, they thought the trach might be able to be removed. And, although her lungs were trashed, in time they believed her lung tissue too could potentially repair itself. As for her short stature and failure to thrive . . . well, they just didn't know. Most assuredly, some of it was caused from the early and continual insults to her body: the vomiting, the lack of nutrition, and whatever happened prior to birth. The genetics report they had run would not be back for a month or two, but they let us know she had passed through all the "known syndromes" because of her mental acuity and ability to keep up with the milestones and development. And so she did not match any of them.

When we returned home from Mayo, things became somewhat better. Within six weeks of our being back, Tayt had gained over four pounds and was beginning to lose the elf-like quality that had plagued her throughout her life. It is hard not to look like an elf when you are starving. Moreover, her ears, which were already bent from prematurity, had in most of the NICUs been taped back (and anyway, in the others, the various tubes strapped around her head had pushed them down), the effect of this having been given no thought.

Although she began to look more like a human being, she continued to be plagued with numerous bouts of pneumonia, and frequent hospitalizations, which were now at another hospital closer to us. We had found a new ENT, which was our go-to for the basics and immediate care in our area, but we were now prepping her for moving on, getting surgery, and starting on the road to being free from the trach that ruled our lives. To be free of the trach meant that the simplest of things could be done. We could hire a sitter on a Saturday night; she could take a bath; we could go on vacation; she could go to the grocery store. It would mean fewer hospitalizations, attending a normal school, playing outdoors, going swimming. It was then I vowed that as soon as Tayt got her trach out we were going to travel. Nothing was going to keep us home once she was free of it.

The surgeon had told us to go home and take care of the things that we could. She needed several "pre-surgical procedures" for the major reconstruction to be successful. There were three main items on that list: she needed to have her tonsils and adenoids removed, she needed to work up the muscles of her lungs, and she needed learn to use her mouth to breathe. We were told of a Passy Muir valve. This was a cap that was placed directly over the trach: allowing Tayt to take oxygen in through the trach, but to exhale through her mouth. It would also give her the ability to talk. When we first put the valve on, it made her so angry she would rip it off. It was uncomfortable and scary for someone who didn't even know what her mouth was for, much less how to use it. Slowly we would place it on when she wasn't looking, and we would try to increase the time that she could keep it there. Initially she couldn't have it on for more than a second or two without it causing the same vomiting, coughing, and retching we had fought so hard to eliminate.

Two weeks after we came home, I placed the valve on the trach and something miraculous happened—and I don't use that word lightly. Tayt looked around the room, surprised. It was like she finally realized she could breathe through her mouth; she finally realized what it was for, and how to control the flow of air through it. A calm came over her, and she turned to me and, in the calmest, most uneventful manner, she made a noise. It wasn't a retching noise, a vomiting noise, or even the smacking noise that she had learned to make to get my attention. It was almost like a hum. It was a noise that plays over and again in my mind to this day. She uttered her first sound; a sound so beautiful and unassuming, yet the look of elation on my face must have been a look Tayt had not yet seen. I think she was completely and utterly taken off guard. There we sat, just the two of us, both astonished by the other's actions and capabilities. For a minute neither of us made a noise, and then she attempted it again. This time she tried to make the noise intentionally. It came out a little less muffled, a little louder; and, with the force of her try, the valve shot across the room. We looked at each other in amazement and broke out into laughter.

We all spent the entire afternoon crying tears of joy. Putting on the valve and having it inevitably shoot off: it was a new parlor trick. It was a true miracle to me. You are always excited to hear your child's first words; not their first *sounds*. I had long since given up on hearing her voice, or forgot that she was even supposed to have one, and here she was: talking, making noise. She had perfected it in her brain and now was able to vocalize for those around her.

Things at home were at long last on a path that was somewhat normal. Colin and I had finally found a piece of happiness; a little piece—an island, if you will—of happiness. If we had become isolated during the terrible times, then we full-on barricaded ourselves in come the good ones. We almost didn't want to share the bits of normalcy.

Finally, too, we had been able to find a steady day nurse. We had recently lost one who we thought would last a while, and who had been working five days a week. But along came Sherrie, who had moved here from Louisiana. And if the Passy Muir had changed our lives, then Sherrie was on the podium alongside it. Her presence and stability allowed me to open up, to gain a little independence, to let go of a lot of control, and to gain a really amazingly great friend all at the same time. By the time Sherrie started with us, I had been left high and dry more times than I could count. But Sherrie would end up staying with us for over two years.

Once Tayt began putting on weight, she became so much stronger and had so much more energy, both mentally and physically. Her newfound way to communicate breathed new life into our home. I exhaled this fresh oxygen, inhaled again, and felt ready to take on the world. Tayt and I could do this. She was going to be "normal"; she was going to one day stand on her own; and I was going to push her hard enough to do that. The nurses in the past had come and gone, most staying only a week; most looking at me disapprovingly when I refused to pick Tayt up when she cried, when I refused to stop massaging her foot, or forced her to crawl to get what it was that she wanted. She had not yet learned to walk at the age of thirteen months, but she had developed the ability to scoot. She could take one leg and scoop it behind her, and then literally propel herself off of the ground to move anywhere she wanted to go.

As Joe had taught me, I made her spend time on her stomach—something she hated. The trach, combined with being on her stomach, would cause her to choke and cry and start with her vomiting routine. But I knew she needed the tummy time. It was hard to watch her get herself so worked up, but I knew that the discomfort of being on her stomach would end. But the development that she would miss from *not* being on her stomach? That would not return. It was now or never. I know there were several nurses who thought that I was being unrealistic; I was pushing her beyond her capabilities; I was being mean, or insensitive. But I still look at her to this day and know in my heart that, if I had let her be—if I had picked her up and moved her from room to room, allowed her not to be on her stomach, catered to her whims as the nurses had thought I should—she would no doubt have cerebral palsy. Maybe a mild case, but she would.

I never pitied her. I still don't pity her. She is a beautiful, smart, charming, fun, and amazing person, and if I had failed to see that, failed to bring that to the surface, that would have been my greatest failing as a parent. I am proudest of myself for having the strength to push and believe in her—medically, emotionally, and physically. God gave her to me for a reason; she picked me for a reason. I took that role very seriously, and still do. Her story is still unfolding, but she has the power to take hardships, challenges, and adversity head-on—not cower from them, or think that she can't do it.

The parade of nurses in and out of our home was almost comical to watch. Colin would come back from work and I would begin telling him of the new nurse who came that day. If you ever enjoyed the late-seventies show *Three's Company*, we began naming the nurses, as Jack Tripper had ("The Lovely Lolita", "Boom Boom Betty"). We named them that, slightly to keep them straight, though mostly in order to laugh at a situation that if not laughed at could make you cry. Though, as I say, the one constant who came to change our world was Sherrie.

It got to the point where Tayt was getting ready to walk. She was so fearful, and most of her movements, although much improved, were still immature. That was something that had not changed. Joe finally said, "If we don't get her up and walking soon, we are giving time for her brain to learn wrong movement patterns. We are giving the brain an opportunity to not bridge the damage that she has sustained." Joe told me that, to overcome it, I had to stand her up and back away. She needed to learn the ability to react to a fall, to brace herself, to develop the natural reflexes that were missing. Tayt went from taking one cautious step . . . to taking two . . . and within three weeks, she was walking—not with an awkward gait; not with any ticks, nor with hesitation. She was walking fluidly; walking like any other fourteen month old. In time, she would walk, run, and play with the ease of any other child.

With the miracle effects of the J-tube—those of gaining weight, and keeping food down—came the misery of the tube itself. As with everything in Tayt's world, every silver lining has a cloud. And the J-tube, while a lifesaver, was also somewhat of a curse. The initial G-tube was a permanent button that was surgically placed, but the J-tube was merely an extension of the G-tube. It was not permanent, and it could come out at any time. It also became clogged, and it was a really hard thing to maintain. Every time the J-tube became clogged it required a trip to the hospital, and by extension our scheduling the radiologist to reinsert it; and, although Tayt's issues were way more important than the accumulation of radiation, my heart was nevertheless sick that she was being exposed to carcinogenic rays so frequently.

We were also told that, at some point, she could develop infections that would be life-threatening and which were impervious to antibiotics, and so in an attempt to eradicate infection from the get-go, we had to give her things like Omnicef and Cipro (those of us who lived through the "anthrax attack" will remember Cipro as the only thing that would save us!). About three weeks after we got home from Mayo, her J-tube became clogged, in what would be the first in a series of similar incidents. The Cipro, which had small particles, would clog the J-tube whenever it was administered.

At the time, despite knowing it was crazy, I was hell-bent on having another baby. In fact, from the time that we had Taytem—literally three weeks later, stressing over how she was not going to live —I was on the warpath to have another child. Maybe because I hadn't yet gotten to bring her home; though probably just because I had always wanted a ton of babies. I wanted at least six children. Colin knew that from the beginning, but I suppose he always hoped that I would change my mind, or that he would change his own.

*

I remember, right after he was diagnosed with pancreatic cancer and his numbers were coming back well, there was a time when we believed that he was going to be cured. He admitted to me that he wanted to have more children. He promised me that he was going to get healthy and we would try again.

*

I wanted another baby, but was crazy concerned about having more problems. So when we went in to have the J-tube reinserted with the assistance of an x-ray, I was too scared to go in with Tayt. Instead I sent my mother. I sat out in the hallway: knowing, because we had been through this several times, that the procedure should take only about ten minutes. It was easy for any seasoned radiologist, and by the looks of the one on call, he was. I sat in the hallway on my cell phone, making appointments and taking care of things around the house, but when too much time had passed and she still wasn't out, I knew that something that was so routine and so simple was not going the way it should. At the time when the doors should have been being opened and doctors should have been bringing Tayt to me, my mother came out of the exam room, looking anguished. I panicked. "What is going on?!" The expression on her face told me that something had gone wrong, terribly wrong. Only Tayt could go through a procedure that seems totally simple, and end up with my mother shaking and near tears.

"They lost the tube inside of her."

"They did what?"

"He lost the tube inside Taytem."

"What does that mean?! How on earth does that happen?!"

I started to run past her, to find out what they had done to her now.

As I flew into the exam room, there lay Taytem, unable to speak. They had removed her Passy Muir valve, the one thing that allowed her to use her voice. Three women I had never met were holding her down with quite some force. This little creature was being held down, while this man was standing over, her pushing something into her. Her face was red, and she was so upset that she was choking on her own saliva. The radiologist was looking at me now.

"We are having a hard time getting it in."

That was his explanation of what had happened: "a hard time".

"As I was doing the procedure," he continued, "I had one of the nurses holding onto the tube, but it split in half and now half of the tube is loose inside her."

I could tell that he was choosing his words very carefully, but I just stared at him in disbelief.

"How did it 'break in half'?"

"Well, I went to guide it and it got too close to the tool and it split."

"Mom, what happened in here? You were in here—what happened?"

"He was putting the tube in, and all I heard was 'Oh shit!' and then 'This has never happened before'."

"I never said that," he shot back. "I never said any of that."

My stomach felt sick as he started to tell me our options.

"Well, we can go in and I can try to 'snag' it, but that could rupture her bowel and she could bleed to death. Or we could just leave it and hope that it passes."

"It passes?"

"That she is able to dispose of it through her feces."

Those were my options. I was either to tell this man to go in and fish out a feeding tube from her bowels, or watch and wait for it to pass. The answer was obvious to me. I picked her up and pushed through the exit and didn't look back until I was in the car, my mother in tow. We sat in silence the whole way home, until I asked:

Did he really say 'Oh shit', Mom?".

She just looked at me in disbelief.

As instructed, I waited thirty-six hours for it to pass. It was not an easy period, because Tayt was dehydrated, trying to recover from the ordeal, tired, worn out, and mentally affected by having been held down and hurt again. After about a day and a half of waiting and worrying, I called Colin at work to tell him that the tube had in fact passed. As I looked at it, I started to wonder what all the hassle was about. This tiny tube would probably never have caused any problems. But the lying, the chaos, the damage to her psyche—that was where the danger in all of this lay. That was where it could have been prevented with a "sorry".

Colin called the radiology department immediately. They told us to come in first thing in the morning, and although they had a full schedule they would squeeze her in.

"You better," Colin said. "You all made the mistake to begin with, and she hasn't had anything to eat in over four days because of it."

The next morning we went to the hospital. There we sat with Tayt, who was lifeless, unresponsive, starving. By this point she couldn't even lift her head. She was writhing in pain as Colin held her. As two hours went by and we sat in the "pre-op" room, occasionally pacing, Colin finally called someone over and started in on them. Our concerns were quickly dismissed, and we were told that, since "we were not on the schedule to begin with", we were lucky that they were squeezing us in.

Colin started talking—well, who am I kidding? *Yelling*—at the top of his lungs:

"You are squeezing US in?! YOU lost a tube in our daughter and are squeezing US in?! YOU have made her go without fluids or food for over forty-eight hours because of YOUR mistake... and YOU are squeezing US in?!

"My mother-in-law caught Dr. Sims lying," he carried on. "'Oops, Oh shit': is that standard in a procedure?! And then he lied about it, and now my baby is dying... do you see her?! Do you not see her dying in front of your eyes... and you are doing US the favor?!"

Colin accompanied Tayt into the exam room. He was not going to let the procedure be done without him present. Finally, after the tube was placed and we were on our way out the door, we were handed a letter, asking us—well, *telling* us, really—that the entire radiology department of Lakeshore General would no longer be treating Taytem. Since the procedure that she needed with the J-tube was "elective", they could by law deny us care, and that was exactly what they were now doing. They hurt her, and we were no longer welcome. The fury of what they did was soon replaced by the fury of the audacity of their response to what they had done. We were now either banned from or intentionally avoiding all of the area specialty hospitals that are equipped to deal with the needs that someone like Taytem requires. We were out on our own—for questioning, for being angry, for speaking up when our child was hurt.

Chapter 13

People say that life is funny. If it is, I suppose it's the hitting-your-funny-bone kind of funny. There is nothing actually funny about going along, feeling in your stride, and then something coming to trip you up. Funny is supposed to mean amusing, something to evoke laughter. It can also mean odd, strange, unexpected. If my life is one thing, it is "funny" in the most unfunny way.

*

Life seemed to be almost returning to normal. Colin and I were letting people back into our secluded world. My friends slowly started calling me again—the ones that I'd kept in sporadic touch with, anyway; and old wounds of not being invited, feelings of hurt and of being left behind, started to fade somewhat. Taytem's problems continued to be an issue, but although the continual "fire drill" never stopped, it got somewhat less.

With things being on the mend after visiting the Mayo Clinic and our family finally seeing a day where we could live a normal, happy, less chaotic existence, Colin and I decided to try IVF to have another child. Since we had not had an easy time getting pregnant, or staying pregnant for that matter, I wanted help with fertility. I'd had enough waiting and crossing my fingers, really, for a lifetime, and just wanted to start to move on. When I found out I was pregnant with our third, I couldn't have been more elated.

Since we did not think that it wasn't a genetic condition that caused Taytem's issues, we assumed that the only problem that we were having was getting pregnant. After having Taytem, and being told that it was not her genetics, our not having found a cause for her issues still left me in doubt. This, added to the failed pregnancy I'd experienced before that, meant I was consumed by the thought of something going wrong. And so we had decided to do IVF, meaning we could test the embryos to give us more assurance.

Moreover, Colin was beginning to work longer hours. To put it into perspective, his work hours when we started out had seen him leave home at eight in the morning and return at half-three in the afternoon. It is amazing how quickly you can become spoiled. That meant that, when his hours increased and he wasn't home until seven, it was a huge adjustment. Tayt's medical situation was becoming less dire; but, with the addition of the pregnancy, I became slightly overwhelmed (and definitely more emotional). I missed him, and was sad that the only time he got to see the kids was on the weekends, since he was leaving before they got up and returning just as I was putting them to bed. As I say, it was a real adjustment.

Our third child was due to arrive in November, but in October Tayt had a terrible cold that started to develop into pneumonia. Although we were no longer welcome in the radiology department of Lakeshore General, her pulmonologist was still on staff there. If there was one person I trusted to truly care about Taytem, and who I knew to have the patience of a saint, it was Dr. Ahman.

I had become very good at monitoring her lung status, and by now probably had as much experience with a stethoscope as a seasoned nurse or doctor. I used to say that I couldn't walk into any room in a hospital and tell you what the patient had, but I *could* tell you within a minute what Taytem had—and I have never been wrong. This time, Taytem was just not bouncing back. She was precisely like that: she would either get better really slowly, or within hours of an illness she would go drastically downhill. On this occasion, she looked like she was near death's door. We still had the oxygen set up at home as a backup, and she still slept with the Pulse Ox monitor on to measure how her body was oxygenating. The readings were horrible. Her breathing was very fast and shallow, and her fever was rapidly increasing. Dr. Ahman did not have clinic hours that day, so he asked us to meet him in the emergency room.

We hopped in the car with Sherrie in tow and arrived at the emergency room. We were quickly escorted into a side room, and an unfamiliar doctor came rushing in.

"We are supposed to be waiting for Dr. Ahman," I said.

By this time my patience, my trust, and my attitude were spent. I didn't have the energy to deal with anyone else. The head resident came in and spoke reassuringly.

"Dr. Ahman is working after hours on an emergency, so we are going to just treat her."

Although I was nervous, I stepped aside, figuring this was just going to be the routine x-ray—antibiotic—home course that we had followed so many times before.

The doctor listened to Taytem's lungs and turned to me.

"She is not getting any oxygen," he said. "It's so tight that her lungs must be completely filled with fluid. We have to go in there immediately and break up the fluid so that she can breathe again."

Sherrie and I looked at each other—thinking the same thing, yet apparently not in any position to disagree with the head of the emergency department. Finally I spoke up.

"I don't think you are right. I know her lungs, but I don't hear any crackling anywhere. I don't hear any pneumonia-type symptoms . . . I think it's more of an asthmatic response."

"I beg to differ," he shot back, as if to say, "How dare you? You aren't a doctor". He told his nurse to get racemic epinephrine and start Taytem's treatment.

As is always the case in any hospital: once the recommended medicine was requested, there was a delay in getting it. When the nurse finally came back in, Tayt by now was listless: on oxygen, red-faced yet with no fever (which was the sure indicator of pneumonia), but clearly in need of something. The nurse put the medicine into the nebulizer cup and started the treatment. Within moments, Taytem looked over at me in panic and started to collapse, her eyes moving erratically from side to side. She was searching for breath, but none was available. Seconds later her lips began to turn blue.

"Stop the treatment!" I was screaming, as I made my way toward her.

The nurse, who apparently was not seeing the same signs as I was, looked back at me, somewhat annoyed by my continual need to be present.

"Stop the treatment!" I shouted, ripping the cup from Tayt's face.

She completely blacked out, her eyes rolling back in her head.

"Do something!" I screamed. "She can't breathe, do something!"

They picked up an oxygen bag and started bagging her. Her oxygen saturations plummeted. When we had come in they had already been at a dangerous eighty-nine; they now read forty-six. She was dying, before my eyes. They were preforming CPR on her, right in front of me. I was escorted from the room, screaming at the top of my lungs:

"You are killing her! What happened?! When I brought her in she was fine! You are killing her!"

Three women literally carried me out (apparently, I was upsetting the other patients). I stood in the hallway after I had calmed myself, looking at her through the peek window. I was angry at myself for not taking my stand. After all the mistakes that had been made, all the times I knew they were wrong yet had not spoken up, I had thought I was past being silent.

I hadn't noticed his presence before, but up behind me came a priest.

"Is that your daughter in there?" he questioned.

Realizing that he was a man of the cloth, I thought it not the right time for sarcasm. (Also, I was too freaked out to even try it.)

"Yes, and she was fine when I brought her in," I said in a barely audible voice, "she was fine when I brought her in and there she is, dying."

"Sometimes things change in an instant, sometimes things are unpredictable, but God is taking care of her, God will make this situation right."

And as quickly as he had appeared, he disappeared.

I looked in the room and realized that they had gotten her stable. Her oxygen saturations had come back up, and she was beginning to breathe on her own.

I rejoined Tayt—never moving more than an inch away from her—while they found her a room. The resident that we had originally spoken to, clearly shaken, had by now come back into the room, and talked with us for what seemed enough time to cover himself. There was no apology, no admittance of wrongdoing; but he was clearly upset and remorseful for not having listened to me.

We ended up staying for a week. Across the initial twenty-four hours, Tayt was in the intensive care unit. She would die in front of me four times that first evening alone, only to be revived on each occasion. And it was in that hospital stay I realized that, even when the buzzers and alarms went off, it was me who would have to be there. After I was awakened repeatedly by her sats plummeting again, I also realized that—no matter how healthy we got Taytem, no matter how much better her medical status got—she would still only be on loan to me. She would always be a sick and fragile child, and I knew that to become close to her, to care about her, to dwell on her, would be the end of me. I had to maintain my distance from her if I was to survive living and being "Tayt's mom".

I still maintain that distance today. If she crawls up in my lap, I am quickly up and doing something to get her off my lap, away from the closeness. I detach myself—not because I don't love her, but because I love her too much. As in the good cop, bad cop scenario, Colin was the opposite. Maybe he knew somewhere deep down that he was not to lose her—she was to lose him. I think he knew his time with her was going to be fleeting, and the only way that she was going to make it in this world was through the encouragement and belief that he afforded her, and his belief in me. I pushed, while he pulled her in. We were the perfect team to make her all she is today.

In November of that year, Matthew came along. He has been the purest joy of the past eight years. His birth made me look ahead; to think that life could be normal. That there could be more to life than hospitals, trachs, sickness, G-tubes, feeding, physical therapy, occupational therapy, weighing Tayt daily. Matthew came along and, after all the stress of the pregnancy, he was absolutely the sweetest surprise since Jake's birth. I would lay on the floor with him for hours, disappear into my room with him, take pictures, just find sheer joy in the absence of his trach, the absence of a feeding tube; his ability to breathe normally, to coo, to drink a bottle: all the things that come so naturally for a baby, and all the things that Taytem could not do.

Taytem's medical issues began to cause us some major financial problems. Her medical insurance was always hard to maneuver. In particular, every time there was a change in insurance of any kind, which there was frequently due to Colin's employer, we would be at risk of losing Sherrie. Colin, who was still a trader, had decided to start a company with Charlie, a good friend of his. Charlie had been something of a mentor to Colin, although he never would admit it. He began trading at the same time as Colin and they had both cut their teeth as clerks. Charlie had started trading slightly quicker than Colin, and had instantly got it. He was a quick learner, less risky, and somewhat more serious, so when Charlie decided to start up his own company—which would grow to an empire—he asked Colin to come along to help. But, after Colin had exploded on several of the clerks (albeit not for no reason), Charlie had given Colin the option of leaving or attending anger management classes. I ignored this; I thought it would go away.

With every move of the insurance, it would send me into a panic. This is probably what caused Colin—so mild-natured, so calm, so NOT excitable—to freak out, thinking, *I have to go home and tell Julie that it's switching again?!* On the very last insurance change that he had with his company, I got on the phone and gave the kid at Colin's work a piece of my mind. At the time—probably because I wasn't listening, probably because of Tayt's need for cover—I didn't care: I gave the new kid, who I thought was just in charge of the human resources, my three cents. When I was done, I hung up and looked over at Colin, who had a look of both relief and fear on his face. At the time, he never told me that this man was not just the HR guy but one of his bosses. I think he knew in his heart that I might have just talked us out of his job.

Colin showed up for work one day to find that his key card didn't function. He checked in at the desk to find out what the problem was, only to get Charlie on the phone saying, "Oh, it's just a mistake; come on up". He was then greeted at the door by Charlie and two lawyers, who took him to a room where he learned of his dismissal. Now Colin had no job; we had a new house we couldn't afford; we had Taytem, who we never could afford; and a six-week-old baby.

Colin was told to look over the dismissal package, which he had exactly twenty-four hours to accept or he would just be fired. He was given a very generous severance, but he had to agree not to work anywhere else in the next three months, or he would forfeit the severance money.

This meant he was at home with me for three months. He knew all he had to do was go back down to the floor of the trade building and someone would love to snatch him up. The Board of Trade was like a man's club where everyone knew everyone else. If you had a good reputation, losing one job would quickly be followed by finding another within a matter of days (if not minutes). Colin was admired on the trading floor. The problem was that, although finding a new position would not be a challenge, the severance package came with the stipulation that he could not trade for the following three months. While he waited on the sidelines before jumping back into the job he loved so much, he became withdrawn, depressed, despondent—with good reason. Trading was a distraction for him and it gave him a purpose, so sitting it out was difficult. I understood that he felt helpless and wanted to get back on the floor to trade as quickly as possible, but his withdrawal from me and our family for the proceeding months felt personal.

Chapter 14

When Tayt was born, I would insist that there is always a "wizard", meaning the guy behind the curtain who can make real change. Many think of the wizard as the fake who is standing behind the curtain out of fear. I see the wizard as the unassuming man who doesn't want to step into the spotlight and take credit; one who's in it purely for making silent change happen. When Tayt got sick, the "experts"—standing out in front, singing their own praises, giving lectures—had lost touch. Not until we found the true "wizard" behind the scenes—not taking credit for their good doings, just doing good—did we find a way to heal as a family.

Now, I am trying to find the wizard for Colin.

*

As the months went on, life with Taytem became more "normal" again. Her medical issues were more manageable, or I took them more in stride. With Sherrie's addition into my world, I began to go back to work here and there, though nothing serious (teaching personal training classes at the local health club).

We had scheduled Tayt's necessary surgery. She was having her tonsils and adenoids removed as part of the surgery prep, when her ENT in Chicago asked what procedure we were thinking about having done to remove her trach. When I told him how it had been described to me, he told me it was a vocal cord lateralization. It was a procedure where they went in and literally tacked back the vocal cords in order to allow air to pass. He asked me why we had chosen the Mayo Clinic, and why we hadn't decided to just go to Cincinnati to the world-renowned doctor who had developed the procedure, along with hundreds of others like it, and who had written over two hundred and fifty books. I hadn't any idea that the very person that developed, perfected, and taught the procedure was that close to us. He told me that he would contact the office of this man, Dr. Collins, and see if he could get us in to see him.

We finally got in touch with his team, made an appointment, and we were set to go at the end of the month. I had contacted Dr. Thomas, to avoid burning any bridges, and indicated to her that we were going to put things on hold for a while. Because of Tayt's size we going to give her time to recover, to focus on getting stronger and getting better.

When it was time, we hopped in the car, made reservations at some obscure hotel in a rough area outside of Cincinnati, and headed off. Matthew was nine months old, and quite a terror. He was adorable; there was NO mistaking that: puffy cheeks, huge dimples, and a smile that could melt your heart. But he was also so high maintenance. He never slept; I have never known a child to sleep less. And when he cried, it was such a high-pitched sound it actually hurt. He would cry all night long. So, there we were in the car—Taytem, Matthew, Colin and I (Jake stayed behind with my mother)—heading out to meet "the guy". Matthew was very unhappy, we got lost trying to find the hotel, and the tension in the car was mounting quickly. Finally, after the four-hour trip (plus an additional hour spent locating the hotel) we pulled into the parking lot and jumped out of the car. Matthew: getting what he wanted, which was getting out of the car, immediately stopped his incessant screaming and crying. Feeling like a vise had been removed from around our heads, we exhaled, unpacked, and began to get ready for the day ahead of us.

We had arrived in Cincinnati for our day of back-to-back appointments. Tayt was scheduled for a scope of her throat, her lungs, her esophagus, and more genetic testing. The tests were performed by colleagues of Dr. Collins; in fact, we had yet to meet him. The colleagues were all very nice, and were completely underwhelmed by her characteristics, and unimpressed by her size or her history. Nothing about her stood out to them. We were there for one reason and one reason only: her throat.

Everyone we met seemed to agree that she would probably be a great candidate for the vocal cord lateralization. Except, that was, for the pulmonologist. He was unsure whether Taytem could handle the surgery. With her history of recurrent pneumonia, and after having read the detailed history and findings from Dr. Thomas, he warned us that, if we went ahead with the surgery, we were exposing Taytem to the risk of completely ruining her lungs—in effect, killing her. We could run the risk of destroying her lungs through aspiration.

(Aspiration is what most of us call when food or liquid goes "down the wrong pipe". It is when what you eat or drink goes down your windpipe instead of your esophagus. It can lead to bacterial buildup in the lungs or pockets of infection, which, over time, can lead to lung failure and death.) We also risked getting to the point where it would be impossible for her to eat. These were the decisions we were faced with. It was never a minor decision, like "Should we put her in private or public school?" It was "Should we put her through major surgery and run the risk of potentially killing her? Or do we just let her have a trach for life?"

We were summoned back to the office to meet with the team. They all gave their exact findings, what they meant, and their recommendations. We sat there, wishing they would get to the point more quickly and just tell us what their conclusion was. When it came to the last expert, Dr. Woll, the room was quiet. Whatever his recommendation was, whatever his findings were, would sway exactly how we would proceed; influence exactly what Tayt's life would be going forward.

"What I found," he said, "went against everything I assumed I would. We found absolutely no evidence that she was in any way aspirating any food. Not only am I shocked by the findings, because I was sure that she was having trouble swallowing—which would cause the cough that you describe throughout her history; and, with the amount of times you describe her throwing up, naturally I would expect to find aspiration—but in her case there was none." As he talked he became more enthusiastic, almost breaking into a smile, and you could see that a smile was not his norm. "So, if the decision were up to me, if it was my daughter, I would go ahead with the surgery. I think her odds of it being successful are very good. I don't think she'll have any problems with aspirating. I can't promise that nothing else will be a problem, but in my experience, the lungs will not be an issue."

For the first time in our long journey with Taytem, since the day I laid eyes on her at Children's Hospital so long before, I believed in the possibility that she might live a normal life. Not "normal" by everyone else's standards, but a life without seclusion, a life of being able to go places, sleepovers, swimming, showers . . . a life of being able to be like everyone else.

They wanted to schedule her for surgery for two weeks after our visit, in the early spring when cold and flu season was over. We were told how, after she had the surgery, she would not be able to wear the Passy Muir valve or to talk for at least a week while the stent was in. They would do the surgery, then we would return home. Two weeks after that, we would then go back to try to decannulate.

Even the very word *decannulate* lifted my soul. To even consider the possibility that we would be free from the trach—to dare to dream—well, it was truly a joy unlike any other.

"Her voice will be fine, won't it? I mean, she won't lose it?" was the last question I asked on the way out of the room as we were leaving.

"No, she will not lose her voice. It will be more 'airy' or wispy, but she will not lose it. She will still be able to talk."

Two weeks later, we were on our way to surgery. I was told that the procedure would only last a day and that we would be on our way back home within forty-eight hours, so I left Matthew and Jake with my mother. Colin, who had already taken way too much time off, had to return to work. After losing his last position, he had decided to go out on his own and began trading on the floor for himself. His new position gave him more control, but it also meant that he was trading on his own without a net. We departed for Cincinnati at two a.m., planning to be there by eight that morning. I was on the road for about an hour—not even through Chicago—when I realized that the major interstate leading to Cincinnati had been completely shut down. The road was totally closed: hundreds of cars, no one moving. Figuring that this was one of the biggest days of Tayt's and my life, I was in a panic. We sat on that highway for two hours, not moving a single inch, until they finally opened the road up again. I made great time, yet nevertheless arrived frantic, crazed, and still an hour late: running with her to make sure that her space did not get filled.

The team brought her back into pre-op, where we went through the usual questions. They gave her a breathing treatment and we waited our turn. Generally, when they brought Taytem for surgery, they would usher us into the room wherein they administered the anesthesia. They always gave the same speech: "Don't be alarmed; when the medicine is administered, she will look a little scary; her eyes might roll back into her head and she might be unresponsive. Don't worry about it; she will be fine". I was in tears. I was putting Tayt's whole life in their hands. I was giving her future to another human being, Dr. Collins. He came out, and for the first time I met "the guy". Up until now, he had only consulted. I had heard all about him, about what he would do, about what he would allow, but he had never been available to be there during the meetings. He stood around five feet six inches tall, gray hair, in scrubs and a hat. He came right up to me, patted me on the shoulder, and said, "She will be in good hands; she'll be fine, I promise".

After exactly three hours, I was summoned to the conference room. I entered from the waiting room, whereas the doctors would enter from the operating room. The room was tiny, but had a phone plus a light for viewing x-rays. It was very cold. I sat and waited until Dr. Collins walked through the door. He told me that it had all gone well. They were going to move her to a room overnight and he would come check on her before we left. He was sure that it was a success, and that she would be great. He told me to schedule an appointment for decannulation, and that he would see us then; and, if we needed anything, to call his office.

When we returned home and tried to carry on life as normal, it was not easy. The anticipation of having a whole Tayt—no nursing, no trach—was too much, almost unreal.

On the Thursday morning exactly two weeks after the surgery, we headed back to Cincinnati. We arrived just in time to make it for our appointment. They took her into the treatment room, just as before, and within ten minutes they came back. I had become very good at reading faces and knowing which way a conversation was going to turn. I could see that there was no elation on their faces, no enjoyment in what they were about to say. The conclusion of the procedure that she had just endured was not what anyone had planned, nor what I had wanted to hear: it was not a success. The tiny space they had created by tying back her vocal cord didn't allow enough room for her to breathe without the trach. I was called into a small room to discuss options.

I jutted forward in my seat a little. "What would that mean for her, for her voice?"

"Her voice will be slightly more raspy."

"She won't lose it though, she won't lose her voice?"

"No she will not lose her voice."

We had two options: letting her live with a permanent trach, or giving the follow-up surgery a shot. We had come this far, gone through so many hoops—what choice did I possibly have? I had promised myself at the very start of this course with Dr. Collins that I would have to give up control and I would have to trust someone.

"How soon could we do this?"

"We can go back in there and finish the other one right now."

I looked at my watch, only to realize that Colin was in the middle of the trading day, on the floor. If I called to consult him, they would have to page him, and I didn't really think that there was a question as to what to do.

"Go do it," I answered with more certainty than I had answered to anything. At this point, there was no turning back, no giving up. There was no way that I was going to go home defeated, having not given it every shot.

After three more hours, Tayt was done. I met her in the recovery room, her little body looking so fragile. By this point she had undergone over two dozen surgeries. Over the years I have lost track, but back then I used to count the number of surgeries and procedures: wearing them like a badge to my own refusal to give up, my belief in what they were telling me, my determination to make her whole. As I sat there in the recovery room this time, I saw a little creature who I loved with every part of my being. I would have given my life for her.

We stayed overnight. Tayt was not happy to wake up and find that her throat had been cut again. All the healing of the past two weeks was undone. The drainage tube remained, and the gift of her newly acquired voice was taken from her.

I was caught completely off guard when we got home from Tayt's second surgery to find that I was six weeks pregnant. (That's how unobservant I was—I'd had no idea that I was even pregnant!)

I went in for the initial ultrasound. After I saw the heartbeat, I was relieved that there was a child with a beating heart growing inside of me. A nurse came in to do the final assessment, blood pressure, etc.

"Oh," she noted, "it looks here like your due date is 11 September—that's my birthdate."

I felt a little sick: both because of my extreme morning sickness and because, living in a post-9/11 era, the date—which is, of course, just a date—made my body feel like something was going to go wrong. I felt like it was just a sign of bad things to come, an omen. I shrugged it off as just a reaction to everything that was going on in my world, the hormones surging through my body, the aftermath of Taytem's birth and surgeries. After all, I had had Matthew successfully and without issues. Surely Taytem was an isolated incident.

Being pregnant was such an incredibly happy thing for me. I loved it, and couldn't be more excited—but the fear and sheer panic that would ensue after the initial confirmation was overwhelming. So, two weeks later, when it was time for us to return to Cincinnati with Taytem to try for decannulation—the final try, the last resort—I couldn't go. Not because the doctor said that I couldn't, but because after the failed pregnancies of the past and Taytem's issues, I just couldn't find it within me to justify the trip, the stress, the drive, the lack of sleep. I'm sure too that, partly, I couldn't stand the thought of being there all by myself if it didn't work. If they tried to take that trach out again and weren't successful, I didn't think my heart could take that kind of disappointment. So Colin ended up going.

Following an overnight stay in Indianapolis, Tayt's appointment was scheduled for nine a.m. I'd like to say I waited patiently, yet I'm sure I did anything but that. At four p.m., I got the call. Colin was on the other end of the phone.

"It worked, Jules, the trach is out. She's breathing fine without it. It worked."

I stood there, silently crying. The stress of three long years, disbelief, excitement, a little remorse at putting the baby I didn't know yet above being there in this moment for Tayt—and, just as importantly, for Colin. I wanted so badly to be there: to hug him, to cry with him, to smile with him, to savor the very moment with him. The relief I felt, the sheer joy I felt, was not the same transmitted through the phone.

"I'm going to get food," he continued, "and I'm leaving her with the nurses for now. She will be fine. They all love her, she's smiling, she's happy."

"Is she worried? Having a hard time? Freaked out?"

"No, she's good. I'm tired, worn out; we have to be here overnight, so I am going to go catch dinner and then head to bed . . . Jules? . . . She's good, Jules, the trach is gone and she's good. Jules, I promise, she's good. We're coming home without a trach. I will call you later."

When they got home, Taytem ran out of the car toward me. She had a huge bandage over the trach site, but that was it. It was like I was meeting her for the first time, as if we had adopted a new child.

There were balloons everywhere; it was like a huge birthday party. I was so ill with morning sickness that I was barely keeping myself upright; but there she stood: Taytem, without a trach. We all stood in that front room, Colin looking so tired, me looking green around the gills, and Tayt looking trach-less and happy.

As in all of my previous pregnancies, I became an obsessive freak. I demanded ultrasounds every week to make sure that, if this baby was behind even slightly in growth, we addressed it immediately. I was as sick as I had been with all the others, but there was something about the due date being on 11 September that I still just couldn't get past. I went in faithfully every week for an ultrasound, and, up until the fifteenth week, everything was right on schedule. My OB-GYN, who had stood at my side throughout everything to date, was dealing with her own issues. I hadn't seen her in weeks. I would see the midwife, the nurse practitioner, others from more specialties than I knew existed—but no Dr. Yaney. On the fifteenth-week ultrasound, the nurse practitioner measured the baby and concluded that he was at fourteen weeks' growth. A red flag went up in my mind. With all the fears and doubts that I had about the birthdate, and the pregnancy having been a surprise, it was too much of a coincidence in my head. I asked for the NP to relay the message to Dr. Yaney that I felt something was wrong. I waited all afternoon, but there was no phone call. She finally called the next day. Her voice barely audible, she told me that she had looked at the ultrasound and that I didn't have a reason to worry; everything looked perfectly fine. She understood my concerns, but different people measure things differently and the difference of a week meant nothing.

After two weeks of putting it out of my mind and shrugging it off as just a bad measurement and nothing to worry about, I showed up for my level two ultrasound. I laid down on the bed and the woman started the scan. I kept looking at her: trying to read her expression, trying to figure out what she was seeing, trying to see the monitor to look at the measurements. She turned to me, no alarm in her demeanor, and said that she was going to take the results to the doctor and have him go over it on his own. Again, no flags went up.

Not long after, in walked Dr. Tanner, who was not the regular doctor that I was used to seeing.

"Hi there. I wanted to go over the results with you." As he was talking, in walked another woman: not wearing a coat, and with no telltale signs that she was even in the medical field. "I don't know how to say this—it is never easy, so I am just going to have to say it. The ultrasound is showing that there is an enormous amount of fluid on the brain. Let me show you what I am seeing." He turned the monitor toward me to point out the brain structure. "This part here—you see how it is transparent? That clear area should be gray matter. The fluid has stunted the growth of the brain. The fluid through this section here—" the mouse shot over to a structure of the brain—"should be less than ten, but it's twenty-two."

"What does that mean?"

"That means that there is probably something going on. There's probably some underlying condition causing the brain to not develop correctly."

"Well, what are the odds that this is just nothing?"

I looked at him, pleading for him to be straight with me. I was looking for him to be brutally honest.

"I don't think there is any way that this is nothing. Something like this points to severe mental retardation at best—maybe not even being able to survive."

"Well, how do we know?"

"We can do an amniocentesis right now to determine if it is chromosomal, if you'd like," he offered.

"Okay, let's do it," I said, more definitively than I had answered many things before. Dr. Tanner walked out of the room to prepare for the procedure and his nurse stayed behind. She laid the tools out next to me on the metal table, just so; but when the doctor entered to begin, I couldn't breathe. It was like the air had been sucked out of the room and there was none left for me.

"Wait, wait . . . I can't do this. It doesn't matter; it just doesn't matter. I had an amnio with my daughter—it came back fine, but even her ultrasound was normal. What you showed me: it doesn't matter what the amnio shows. I can't go through with it this time; I can't do it again; I can't live through this again." I literally jumped up from the table at this point.

"I completely understand. If you change your mind and you'd like to have the amnio run, please just call the office. I know this was a huge shock, so you will need some time to process it and talk to your husband. Whenever you are ready and have made a decision about how you would like to proceed, please just call and make an appointment."

I sat alone in that room for just a moment before heading out the door and to the elevator. The problem was, this was not a shock. I was not completely taken by surprise. I'd known from the beginning that this was not right—that there was something wrong. Waiting for the elevator, I almost felt justified, in a way I can't describe. I was more angry than shocked. I was gritting my teeth, cursing God—but without even the energy to curse Him.

I called Colin when I got to the car.

"Colin . . ." I broke off because I couldn't even pull myself together enough to get out what I needed to tell him. I couldn't bring myself to tell him the horror of the ultrasound that I had just witnessed. "It's the baby . . . there's no brain, Colin; this baby has something wrong too, and he has no brain."

There was silence on the other end. I could feel his regret at not being next to me, not being able to be there during the incredibly devastating news.

"I'm going to leave now," he said. "I can be home by two. Just sit tight. What did they say? No, never mind, you can tell me when I get home. Just hold on Julie, remember what happened with Taytem? Maybe they are wrong, Julie; maybe they are wrong again . . . just try to hold on, okay?" Then a pause. "Okay, I will see you in a couple of hours. I love you, Julie. This will be fine, we will be fine. I love you. I have to go or I'll miss the train." I stood holding the cell phone in my hand, not realizing that he was no longer at the other end, perhaps needing to linger just a bit longer to feel connected.

When Colin came home, I took one look at him and just buried my face in his chest. I wanted to crawl inside his skin—just settle and hide there, never come out, never deal with any of this. We decided that, as soon as the kids went to bed, we would discuss what the doctors had concluded, what they had shown me, what they had seen on the ultrasound. The only thing that I could say at the time was, "It's done, Colin. It's done".

After everyone was finally in bed, I told Colin how I had seen the missing gray matter and the fluid on the ultrasound. I'd had proof laid out in front of me that told me what was going on. It wasn't like with Taytem: where they could only tell us she was small, yet they gave us no definitive reason to believe that she was not okay.

Colin hadn't seen it coming any more than the doctors had. He was still holding onto blind faith; still believing they could be wrong, and this baby could be fine. He wasn't sitting in that room, seeing what I had seen. He believed that everything would be alright. He doubted my instinct that something was wrong from the beginning; believed that I was just being paranoid. No matter what I said to him, he had this expression of incredulous disbelief. The follow-up appointment was scheduled for the next day, so as we turned out the lights, he said,

"We'll talk about this again tomorrow after we see the doctor."

The next morning, we took off in the Jeep. We drove directly to the ultrasound appointment and met with the doctor. Within the first five minutes of the ultrasound, Colin saw exactly what I was shown, and was told exactly what I had been told. Then we were ushered off into the conference room.

"So," the doctor started, "I can give you both as much time as you need to make a decision."

"So your opinion is that this is not just 'nothing', and that there is no way this baby could be born completely fine, without any brain damage?" I asked him, so Colin could hear what I had already come to terms with.

"In my opinion, this baby would make it to birth with no brain capacity at all, at best. There is NO way that this is not the symptom of something much larger," he replied.

"Then there is no decision to be made. I would like to terminate this pregnancy. I don't want to continue on with it. How soon can we have this done? I would like Dr. Matthews to do it, but I want it done immediately. I don't want to wait any more than a day or two."

"Of course, I completely understand. I would do the same thing." He called to the front and had it set up to be done three days from then. We left the office, and I almost already felt like I wasn't pregnant anymore. I had convinced myself—sitting in that room, making the decision that I did—that I was no longer pregnant, and the baby that I was carrying was no longer alive. We pulled over to fill the gas tank, and as Colin hopped out I reached into the glove compartment to find an old and forgotten pack of cigarettes that I had from years past. I took one from the box, put it to my lips, lit it, and took a deep breath in. It felt like defiance, and tasted bitter; but no more bitter than my heart felt in that moment. I needed to feel like I didn't care—like it wasn't ever real to begin with; that the baby was just a figment of my imagination from the start—in order to live with what was happening.

We went in the following day for the "prep work". I had no idea what that meant, having never fathomed that I would be in this position. Colin and I showed up at nine for the appointment, at the start of which two women who were new to us brought us into the conference room and asked if they could ask some questions. Although all I wanted was for this to be over, I knew that avoiding them was not going to speed anything up. They turned out to be the geneticists, and they wanted to ask me about risk exposure, previous pregnancies, the problems with this one, normal pregnancies.

I was extremely vague in my answering, which I knew was throwing Colin for a loop. I had never passed up an opportunity to talk about Taytem, but I didn't want to make any such connection with this baby. I felt that if we made any connection that this would be my fault. I knew that if we found a link between this baby and our other children, not only would I feel absolutely responsible for the pain of this baby and ending its life, but I knew that I could never in good conscience try for another. So I refused to give them all the pieces to the puzzle.

After our interview, yet another doctor I had never seen entered the room (although, soon afterward, I would come to refer to him as "the finisher"). He came in and described to me how the entire process would go. Hearing it laid out in detail contained some of the hardest phrases and sentences that I have ever had to digest. When he finished, I wasn't sure how I was going to go through with all of it. I hesitate even now, writing this, and have spared these details from even my closest of friends. In fact, I have not talked about it—even with my mother. The details that follow made me reevaluate my own humanity, reevaluate God, and search myself for forgiveness: a forgiveness that I will never find. I fear reliving it myself, going through it again mentally. It makes me watch shows that go on and on about ending the potential for "late-term abortions" and sit in disbelief, because *Who in their right mind would go through with a procedure so immensely horrible, just because they don't want a baby?* These "late-term abortions" are there to be done purely for medical reasons. Those who *choose* to have them never forgive themselves, nor get over it. In the same sense, if I did not make the decision I had, I would never have forgiven myself for allowing a baby to be born whose sole purpose was to suffer needlessly. The features of the man who told me what the next hour or two of my life would entail were in no way remarkable; but his face, the way that he walked and talked, are all burned into my memory—like a bad dream that you just can't forget or get over. He reminded me of every bad-guy character in every movie that I had ever seen up till then. The finisher: the guy who comes in and does the dirty work that no one else finds themselves capable of doing. He came in the final hour to do things that the other doctors obviously would not do. His name was not on any business card, any office, or any door.

"In order to perform the procedure that you are signed up for tomorrow, I am going to need to insert an ultrasound-guided needle into your abdomen and give the fetus some medication that will make the heart stop beating." In sheer horror, I looked at Colin, thinking *Did he just say what I think he said? Can this be real? Please make him take that back* . . . Colin looked as if he didn't really know what to say or do—as if I was being carried off by a wave, and he was incapable of pulling me back without losing himself in it as well. This tide was way too big; it was capable of carrying us both out to sea.

"So," continued the finisher, "if you will follow me into this procedure room, it will only take a couple of minutes for the medication to start working and then you can return home, and the rest of the procedure will be performed tomorrow in the OR."

"Is this really necessary?" Colin had finally snapped out of his daze.

"Well, it's the best way to make sure that we are being humane. We know that the fetus will feel nothing tomorrow."

Here I was, lying on this table, having finally convinced myself that this baby inside me was not really alive, it was *already gone*. I had reconciled it that way—already gone—but as soon as he said "humane" and "will feel nothing" my theory was completely erased. It had been a baby, it was living inside of me, and although God chose it to not have a brain, I was choosing to take its life from it.

I sat on that table, Colin next to me. The doctor inserted that needle, and the most animalistic noise came from my mouth. "It can't hurt that badly," is what he actually then said to me, and with such disdain—as if even he couldn't stand not only his own job, but the decision that I had made and forced him to follow through with. He injected whatever medicine he had to. He then pronounced, "There, we're done. Now, if you just want to wait a minute or two and we can check . . ."

"I think we need to get out of here," Colin broke in.

"Well, there's no way to make sure it worked . . ."

"Then we will have to just believe that it did."

Colin pulled me from the exam table. I was in shock, completely unaware that I was sobbing uncontrollably, with no recollection of having started to cry.

Colin literally held me up as we walked from the clinic. I don't remember anything of the ride home; or anything, in fact, of the ride to the hospital prior. No recollection of who took the kids, who drove, how I woke up, if I showered, if I brushed my teeth. I was numb, in shock; unsure whether I had made the right decision, and incapable of making any other decisions at all. The only thing that I do recall is showing up at the hospital. Back at home, I sat on a bed and waited for the rest of this nightmare to be over. I just wanted it all to be over. Colin tried to hold onto me, to grip my hand, but I wouldn't allow him to touch me or even get close enough to comfort me. I don't know why I was pushing him away. Perhaps, I didn't think myself worthy of any comfort. I didn't recognize at the time that Colin needed MY comfort too. We had both lost someone we loved.

Colin couldn't stand to see my heart broken so many times. So many times in the past, and here we were again. He moved closer, sitting on the bed.

"Don't, please just don't," I said, pushing him away.

"It's okay, Jules, it will be okay."

"I can't do this anymore, Colin. I just want to die. I don't want to live this life anymore. I want to die. I am tired, so tired of it all. I have just killed my child—how can I live with that, Col? How can I ever live with that? I just want to die; I just don't want to do this anymore."

He grabbed me, not saying anything. No fear. No incredulous actions on his part. Just nothing but sheer comfort, sympathy, concern, and love.

He just sat there and held me. (Finally, I had given in and let him hold me.) I let the shield down. I let him in.

"Are we ready?" asked Dr. Matthews, when we had arrived for the procedure the next morning; looking first at me while I refused to make eye contact, then to Colin, who had tears in his eyes also. Colin nodded to him, and they wheeled me down the hall. As I laid my head back Colin was forced to release my hand, and off into the operating room I went. The anesthesiologist came in, saw my face, and knew that whatever conversation he had planned to have with me would be fruitless. It would be a complete waste of breath and more punishing to me than comforting. He knew that it was prudent to get me started and out as soon as possible. He asked me to count to ten, injected the IV with something, and my mind went fuzzy.

I woke up next in recovery. Colin came back to sit by my side, helped me to dress, and held me up as we made our way to the car. I was too groggy even to cry anymore.

For the next couple of months, Colin and I had a hard time relating to one another. He threw himself into coaching Jake's sports, and I spent more time with the kids. We talked about the weather, the kids, the house, but we didn't really talk about anything that mattered.

Matthew was growing up so quickly. I would wake in the morning, take Matthew and Tayt to the basement, and just hang out for hours watching them. By this time, Tayt had had the trach removed and was starting to gain a little bit of weight consistently. Matthew really brought out the happy in her. They were best friends and just had so much fun together.

After the loss of the pregnancy, I needed another life to bring me back. Colin was adamant that it was not a good idea; I think he was mostly scared that he might lose me forever if something went wrong. We were so at odds, still not communicating, really living separate lives. I had begun to not even notice that we barely talked anymore. We would get all the kids in bed, watch television, and then roll our respective ways away from each other.

Tayt's checkup was coming up again soon, and this time, although Colin's stepfather or my mom normally went with me, I decided that I was just going to do this one alone. I left the house at two a.m., leaving Matthew with my mother, knowing that I could be back by eight p.m. The drive was only about four and a half hours—no big deal, and the morning proceeded as any other would. We made it to the appointment just in time for them to bring Tayt back. I talked to the doctors, I carried her to the exam room; they gave her the anesthesia, her eyes rolled back in her head; I walked into the waiting room. After fifteen minutes, I was called for. I was told where she would be, and headed through the doors to where she was. As I was walking down the hall, the code blue alarm was suddenly triggered, and I was quickly being stampeded by medical staff in a rush to answer the call. I had no idea that we were all headed to the same place.

I looked over at where Tayt was waiting, and realized that there was a curtain drawn at her bedside. The blinking lights, the chaos, the screaming "1, 2, 3 . . . 1, 2, 3 . . ."—it was coming from behind her curtain. I walked over, being pushed aside by two or three staff members as I did, only to turn the corner just in time to see Tayt's lifeless little body on the table, naked and blue. Over her head was a nurse with a bag over her mouth performing CPR, and others all around: injecting her IV with things, shouting. I stood for a second, out of body, looking over the scene in complete disbelief. And then came a blood-curdling scream. It was so primal of a scream that it startled even me . . .

"Oh my God! What is this? What is going on?!" The air rushed from my body. "When I brought her in she was fine . . . what did you do? What did you do?! She was *fine*!" I began shaking and screaming. "What did you do to her?! What have you done?! You killed her! She was fine! She was fine! She was fine!"

Finally, one of the larger male staff members came up behind me.

"Mrs. Barth, let's go this way. You have to get out of their way. Here, let's go this way."

He was trying to get me away from the situation, and I was clearly not going. My legs would not have worked even if I was cooperative enough to want to go—which I was not. Another man came up on my other side.

"Mrs. Barth, really, we need you to get out of the way so we can take care of her."

Finally, in a last-ditch effort to escort me away, they picked me up by the arms and began carrying me through the recovery room.

I stayed in the room where they put me until someone raced in.

"She's fine . . . she's fine; she's breathing, Mrs. Barth; she's fine."

I didn't hear it. I couldn't hear it. I needed to fall apart; the past four years was in pieces around me, and I couldn't hear it. I sat still, screaming into my hands,

"You killed her!"

But maybe what I really meant was that I had killed. Maybe I was reliving the procedure of terminating my own child: a reality I had now ignored for the past six months. It all came flooding back. I was no longer able to keep it on the shelf. The jar had broken, and now I was left to look at the mess all around me.

"She's fine," the woman repeated, thinking maybe I hadn't heard her. But in reality, I was not done. I wasn't done letting it out. I needed to scream, to cry, to get out all the poison that I was holding inside.

"Mrs. Barth, she's fine. She's breathing just fine. She was just having an asthma attack. She's fine, I promise you. She's alive; she is fine."

I knew I had to suck it all up and put on an okay face. Not for me, but for them; all of them, the world. I would pick up all those pieces again, find a bigger jar, and stick it back up on the shelf. I sat at Tayt's bedside. As she woke up, I smiled at her. She was cold and coughing and her throat hurt. We stayed just a couple more hours, to ensure she was stable enough to be able to go home. After waiting it out, I jumped back on the road, to return to a home that would never offer me the security that home should.

The drive was uneventful, but my eyes were drooping. I made it home probably on sheer adrenaline and the need to be with Colin; to have him just give me a hug.

He would make it okay. He always made it okay . . .

Chapter 15

As I lifted up the toilet, I imagined a war scene: the ravaging that war creates, the casualties. I pictured Colin there, vomiting—always vomiting. There are many things I have been able to put out of my mind. Many things that I have been able to forget, to not think about, to push to the back of my brain—like the old man in the library, sequestered into a dark space where no one ever goes. But looking into the face of that toilet, I still saw in the crevices the pain and misery of Colin's final months in this house, the continual vomiting and sickness. I know that I had cleaned it a thousand times. I now remember Colin coming down the stairs after chemo, barely able to navigate the stairs; me on the way up, asking "What Colin? What do you need?"—trying my hardest to not seem annoyed, because he looked so awful.

"Nothing, I am just going to get stuff to clean up . . ."

"To clean up what?!"

He looked off balance, somewhere between the third and fourth stairs, head drooping, barely able to speak.

"I threw up and missed the toilet. It's no big deal, I just need something to clean it up."

"Colin, please don't worry about it, go on back upstairs, go back to bed, it's no big deal, I will be up in a minute to clean it up."

At the time, I was already running late for something, getting someone ready to go somewhere; completely forgetting that he was upstairs, suffering, while my life was continuing on as normal.

I put down whatever it was, treaded up the stairs and had to dismantle the toilet quietly. He had vomited so immensely that it had somehow found its way under the hinges in the back—stuck in the crevices, like all the memories of his suffering are now stuck in the crevices of my heart.

As I knelt down in front of the toilet to clean it today, he is long gone, gone for weeks. But the suffering of months, so many months, is left in the crevices of this house, in all of our hearts—incapable of ever being cleaned out. The stains will remain forever, and will continue to creep back in just when we think we got it all cleaned up and there can't be any more left. Fighting cancer is like war: only you have no one to fight, no one to hate, and no one wins.

He was alone. I was standing next to him—but, in this fight, he was so alone. That is why he was so afraid to lose me, to be without me. He didn't even realize that he had been alone for months already.

There will always be something pulling me back to Colin, to our short and wonderful time together. He will never be cleaned from this house.

*

After the incident at Tayt's checkup, there was an unspoken understanding between Colin and I that I would no longer go to Cincinnati on my own. Even the thought of the next checkup would send me into a panic attack.

Following my return, life seemed somehow changed. A new peace came over me—or maybe it was complacency.

I started letting Taytem go to school, enrolling her in the preschool by our home. Knowing she was a little behind, I had held her back a year. Although she was supposed to be in the kindergarten class, I had put her into the 4K the year before. She failed to make more than one day a week at best due to illness, doctor's appointments, or therapies. Following the third bout of pneumonia, I had decided that was enough, and I pulled her from school. However, after returning from Cincinnati, my soul had been tamed; and I realized that, even if I tried to control everything, it still wouldn't make any difference. I knew it was time to let Taytem live her life. I realized that she was a little girl, who we had fought so hard to keep here, and now it was time to let her experience: to let her grow, and to let her live without being put in a bubble. The control wasn't helping. God was going to take her when He was ready, not when I was ready to let her go.

She started back in the 5s program and really began to blossom. She was finally beginning to make new friends, and to talk to people. Before, she had been quiet and reserved. In fact, I am quite sure most observers had just written her off as mentally handicapped. She would sit on the sidelines when children were around; she wouldn't participate or answer—she was just trying to figure it all out. She had become accustomed to being stared at, and she would just look at them and smile. Tayt had no problem with the stares. She didn't take offense. She wasn't angry. Instead she met their gaze with understanding, as if to say "I get it, I don't look the same".

Colin and I had been married at Christmastime. Jake had just turned two when we had finally decided to do it, and so our anniversary always fell on the same weekend of friends' Christmas parties. This particular year, just starting to heal somewhat from the trip to Cincinnati and the loss of our baby boy, our good friends were having a party. Colin and I had not been at odds, just out of sync. We seemed to not be able to meet. Our conversations were choppy, unemotional, schedule-centered—no feelings, no joy, no emotions to be found. So on our anniversary that year, after having such an awful year, Colin and I took off in a limo to go to our friends' party. It was snowing so badly that, had he not already ordered the limo, I'm sure we would have bagged the entire evening.

We sat in the limo. It was odd: considering it felt like years since I had on anything but sweatpants, and it had been a long time since we had any freedom together. After five minutes of really enjoying the silence from leaving the kids behind, I felt a little like Cinderella. I wasn't the type to make a big effort, but we were in this upscale car, all dressed up like royalty, with snow all around (enough of it to make the night look like it were apt for a fairytale). Colin put up the blocker on the limo, to add a little privacy.

"I know we have had a rough year; it has been a really tough year for you—well, for us. I miss you, Jules. I miss talking to you, laughing with you. I don't want this silence to continue."

I started to automatically answer, "What silence?", but found myself for once biting my tongue and listening.

He reached into his jacket and pulled from his pocket a box—a small jewelry box.

"I am so sorry if I have not been there for you; if I haven't been what you needed me to be. I just love you so much, Jules, I love you so much," he said. For the first time in months, I looked right into his eyes. "Here, I bought you this." He handed the box to me. I opened it up and inside was the most unassuming silver cross. Colin was not a really "religious" person; he was never baptized as a child. When Jake was going through his first communion, Colin decided that he wanted not only to be baptized, but to join the church as a formal member with me and our children, and so went through the program alongside Jake. I can't say I wasn't a little baffled. I was brought up and raised Catholic, but clearly I was angered with God's decisions for me. Colin was aware of my feelings, so I was caught off guard. I took the cross from the box and held it up to my face. Looking at Colin, he was waiting for my expression, looking for my approval. "If you look at the back of it, I had it inscribed, see?" He held the cross close to my face, since the car was dimly lit. "'Jake, Taytem, and Matthew.' Do you see how there is an extra arm? I left it blank to let you know that I would like to add to our family. That is where I would like to put the name of another child."

I was speechless. Tears began streaming from my eyes and ran onto the cross. Colin reached up and brushed them away. He held my face in his hands and looked into my eyes as I was sobbing in disbelief.

"Are you sure?" I questioned him.

"Couldn't be more sure."

*

That is a night that I will remember until the day I die. When I miss Colin, or I need to remember who he was and who we were together, that is the night I return to. Sitting in the back of that limo, talking about our future, our children, a life to move on with—that was who we were together.

*

The next couple of months were filled with laughter and good times. Colin and I loved nothing more than each other's company. We enjoyed just going to dinner, having a couple of drinks, planning, dreaming. We dreamed of a day that Taytem would be free from illness; finishing off a house that we just couldn't ever leave alone; having another—hopefully, God willing—healthy child: those were the things that we hoped for When I think of the best times of my life, they always include Colin.

As Col had promised, we began to try for a fourth baby. Once more, we went through fertility treatments: my again having decided that I didn't want to take a chance by simply trying to become pregnant on our own. Our first treatment cycle appeared to be going incredibly well. At the end of it, they had extracted twelve eggs. To make everything even more exciting, all twelve had fertilized. At that point there was just the matter of doing the genetic testing. We decided to have all the embryos tested to make sure that the genetics were in order. Otherwise, it could be a waste to implant them; or, God forbid, risk having another sick child. The testing would take three days, which was how long we needed to wait to implant the embryos.

I got a call from the clinic at about nine p.m.

"Hello, is this Julie Barth?"

"Yes, it is."

"This is the fertility clinic. I just wanted you to know that we just got back the results from the genetic lab. Great news: it looks like there is for sure one genetically perfect embryo, possibly two."

Stunned, I just answered "Okay, thanks" and hung up the phone.

"Who was that?" Colin asked, already annoyed. In Colin's world, no self-aware adult would call another adult's home after six p.m. unless it was an emergency.

"It was the clinic. They say that we have one for sure, and maybe two good embryos to transplant."

"Do you think they got the wrong people?" he questioned, looking startled.

"I don't know . . . weird, huh?"

Yet there I was the next day, as the woman I had spoken with on the phone pulled out my paperwork and showed me that, indeed, it had not been a mistake. We only had one for sure that looked good. The other had one chromosome that they were quite certain looked okay, but they just couldn't get a good enough look at it. One embryo—the one that was perfect—was a girl, and the other was a boy.

"If I implant them both and the boy's chromosomes are not perfect, is it a chromosome that they can live with? Is it vital, or is it just something that will allow them to make it, but with malformations?"

"If you implant them both and the chromosome is not right, the baby will not make it past ten weeks," she answered. "I would implant both of them if I were you. No harm can come from it."

I looked to her in probably the most awkward way, as if asking her, "Do you have any idea who you are talking to? Do you have any idea what I have been through, the childbearing horror I have witnessed?"

I took her advice, said I would implant them both, signed the papers, and was asked to change clothes and get ready. I was brought into a small room where there were five or six people all around. Within moments my legs were spreadeagled, and I was exposed to all of them. I don't know what the male-to-female ratio was, but I do know the two closest to me were men. They were cheering and congratulating themselves, like it was halftime at the Super Bowl. I was so excited, yet a little awestruck that I could sit there, all dignity gone, legs up in the air (facing the door, no less), and I couldn't care less. If it meant that I could have another child, possibly two, then who cared?

Later that month, we found out that we were expecting our fourth and maybe fifth child. My hormone levels were through the roof, so I was sure I was having twins. I knew however, that if it was just one child, it was almost sure to be a girl. The girl was the perfect one, and if only one made it then that meant it was probably the girl. Four weeks later, I returned to hear the heartbeat. It was the beating of one heart. It was a girl.

The rest of the pregnancy were completely and utterly uneventful. Colin and I spent a lot of time at home; a lot of time watching movies, reconnecting. Colin also spent a lot of time at work.

At the end of the nine months, Pippa arrived. I had been booked in for a C-section, and we had had all the appropriate testing, with everything coming back fine. We'd even had one of those 3-D ultrasounds where the whole face was visible. Regardless, I was terrified.

We would be having her in August. Colin entered the room as they began to strap me down. (For anyone who hasn't had a C-section, when they take your arms and strap them down onto the table, it is an incredibly unnerving feeling. You immediately feel a loss of control.) Then they began to administer the anesthesia, and my body went numb.

The procedure itself went very quickly. The relaxed doctor was making idle chitchatting with me, while they had an on-staff neonatologist present just in case something did go wrong. I guess, knowing my history, they didn't want to take any chances; they must have had the same doubts that I did. There was a lot of tugging and pulling; Colin was at my head, also talking to me about trivial nonsense. And then I heard the doctor say "It's a girl," and I heard a cry—not stridor, weak, unable to breathe—but a real, healthy, "unhappy to be here" cry. They whisked her away and put her under the heating lamp.

"There's a small birthmark on her face," I heard the doctor announce. It struck me as odd, but I assumed it was one of those "cover your butt" statements to name the mark so there was no mistaking whether it was caused during delivery or after. While they were cleaning her up, the neonatologist looked her over, and for the second time I heard someone state how she had a birthmark on her cheek.

I began to panic. I was still strapped down, and they were putting me back together. I looked at Colin and asked him to check on her and make sure that everything was okay. He stood in silence, observing as they washed her. After a moment or two, he began to walk back toward me with the strangest look on his face. The blood had drained from his face and his mouth was agape.

"Is she okay?" I whispered, unable to muster the energy to convey how deeply concerned I was come this point. He started to sit down next to me, missed the chair completely, and fainted, right there, passed out on the floor.

The staff quickly went into action, picking him up, placing him in a chair, and wheeling him out into the hallway. I lay stuck on the operating table, the baby nowhere near me, and with no one rushing her my way. The tears began streaming down my face, not having any way to wipe them from my eyes. The doctor looked at me, not knowing what the exchange between Colin and I had been, and whispered, "He will be fine, Colin is going to be fine, they just took him out into the hall. He's up, he just needs some air". All I could think was *If he is so fine, get his ass in here and have him tell me what the hell is wrong with our baby!* Colin finally reentered the room, and as he did the nurse brought Pippa toward me, wrapped in a towel. She handed her to Colin as they untied my arms so I could hold her.

"Is she okay?"

"Yes, she is perfect," Col said as he handed her to me. I blinked, swallowed, prepared myself. As they handed her to me, I saw a tiny birthmark on the side of her cheek. Not the mammoth one that I had envisioned; certainly nothing that had made Colin pass out. It was a tiny, obscure little "angel's kiss".

"She can have that removed, or she just might outgrow it," the doctor commented as she looked down at Pippa.

"She's fine just the way she is. I couldn't care less," I answered.

To this day, when I look at Pippa, I can't see the birthmark. She is perfect and beautiful, mark or no mark. I don't know that I will ever attempt to have it removed. I have come to believe that it's part of who she is. Part of her personality. Part of what makes Pippa Pippa.

I still have no idea what caused Colin to pass out that day in the delivery room. I don't know what came over him—low blood sugar, another mouth to feed, seeing them cutting me open . . .

Chapter 16

White lies are not just the things that we tell to others to spare their feelings. They are little lies we tell to ourselves to keep going. When we aren't honest with ourselves, sometimes it is the only way to make it through.

*

I have several good friends. But one in particular—whom I have always loved for her honesty, her brass, her "realness"—had seen something on television and approached me with it. There was no filter as she proceeded to tell me that she had found out what Taytem had. She had watched some special on the Discovery Channel about dwarfism. The doctors at four accredited hospitals—including Mayo—could not find out what was wrong with Tayt; but here she was, one of my best friends, telling me that my daughter was a dwarf.

I would be lying if I said I wasn't offended by her diagnosis. I was upset—somewhat angry, really. In no way was she trying to hurt me; in fact, I think she thought she was helping me to figure out what was wrong with Taytem. There is this false assumption that, when a child has something that no one else does, that the parents are "dying" to find a diagnosis. But I was happy they hadn't found one for Taytem: I was happy that she didn't "have" anything. I never stuck my head in the sand, or said she was "normal", or that she ever would be normal. But as long as whatever was going on with her didn't have a name, well, I could go on pretending in my own world that she was going to grow up and be like everyone else at some point—some version of "like everyone else", whatever that might be.

I don't think that she truly understood what her comments did to me, the way they profoundly changed my life. Much like you can't unring a bell, the flippant information changed who I was, and who we were as a family, forever...

As the weeks passed, something started changing; I could feel it. I began looking at Taytem differently—like when you come home from vacation and you notice the flaws of your house that you had, for years, walked past. I started noticing that Taytem was different: not different in a "she had a slow start" kind of way, but truly different—made differently from the rest of us. Her bones were smaller; her head was smaller; she wasn't catching up as they predicted she would. She was lagging far behind. In fact, she was falling further and further behind on the growth charts. All the things that I had been able to overlook, I now saw. Moreover, across the next four weeks I would have three separate public encounters whereby complete and utter strangers asked me the same question:

"Are you the family on that Discovery Channel special?"

That same year at Christmas we were at a party with six of our very closest friends (as in high-school, lifelong friends), and as the beer and wine flowed, so did the jokes. Somehow the conversation turned to midget throwing—not malicious, just something about a show that was on television—and our friend Colin was vividly setting the scene: describing it, embellishing it, adding to it, becoming animated, reenacting . . . really getting into it. Suddenly, the room grew very, very quiet. The joking stopped, and everyone hushed. I was completely oblivious to what was going on, and I suppose buzzed enough not to recognize that anything was. I merely thought his recounting was over, no big deal. But within minutes our friend Colin had come over to me: pleading forgiveness, practically on his knees. "Oh my God, Julie, I am so sorry, so, so sorry, I didn't mean anything by what I was saying . . . I didn't mean to offend Colin or you. I just feel so horrible. It's just that I am sorry that I was making fun of midgets right in front of you both." It took several minutes for the conversation to sink in. At the time, Tayt was not more than two years. I stared back at him, and it was almost like a light finally turned on in my brain.

"Taytem's not a midget, Colin . . ."

I was so completely unaware that they all—all of our friends, all the friends standing in that room—knew what I was so oblivious to; what was right in front of me; what I had denied and explained away since she was born. I wrote off that night, that incident, along with countless others over the first several years of Taytem's life.

Colin had returned to work trading for himself after the insurance incident. That, however, had come without a lot of security and benefits, so he took a new position with a trading group and had started working longer hours. One night, when I had gotten everyone in their pajamas, and had already sorted dinner, which was waiting, ready for Colin's return, on the table, I inched toward the computer. I did something that I had sworn so long ago never to do: I punched, into the internet, the diagnosis that my friend Anne had given to Taytem. "Primordial dwarfism" was the search term, and I found only three individual sites. I clicked on the very first one, and up popped Taytem. I shuddered. I literally felt as if I would vomit at that very moment. I don't know why—I don't know if it was five years of fear, or relief, or a mixture. There was a picture of a girl who looked so much like Taytem that she could have been a clone. There were the eyes that I explained as Grandma Barth's; the nose that surely came from my father's mother; the teeth; the small mouth, which I blamed on the feeding tube forming her palate, her feeding issues, and not being able to grow. Everything that defined Taytem, everything that complicated Taytem: there it was, right in front of me.

I continued on, reading about brain aneurysms, precocious puberty, joint dislocation, missing teeth, height estimate. It was all too much. It was like God putting out an instruction manual on our life—a guide to what was going to happen to us throughout our time here. The problems that I had foreseen with Taytem paled in comparison to what I was reading. I could have gone on in denial forever, but now there was no turning back. Not after this. I had to face the reality of who she was, what she was to become; her prognosis.

The issues that I had not foreseen? Now I had seen them. I had to acknowledge it. My world would be forever altered, and the angst grew as the knowledge slowly killed the protective layer I had used. Then, I thought of Colin. How was I going to tell him about it? How would he react? I had not filled him in on *any* of the earlier rumblings—not Anne's diagnosis; not even the random strangers asking me about Taytem. Colin had always been okay with Taytem. No matter who or what she was, he didn't care. He saw in Taytem perfection. He saw a daughter who needed love and shelter and compassion, while I saw her as a project that needed to be molded, shaped, fixed, pushed. The worst thing that I could find out was that she would suffer more—that her prognosis was going to involve more pain.

Although, in that very same moment, something miraculous happened. I realized in that second that I really didn't love her any less; I didn't think any less of her. I thought *more* of her, given what she had endured.

Colin came home just as I finished looking. The shock was still fresh; the tears were still wet. He walked through the door to find me at the desk, my dinner cold, and the kids having put themselves to bed somehow.

"Jules, what's wrong?" He inched closer to me. "What is it?"

"I know what's wrong with Taytem. I know what she has." I turned the monitor toward him.

"That's her, alright."

"I know . . . what do we do?"

"What do you mean?" He looked at me, puzzled.

"Well, I mean . . . what do we do?"

I looked back at him. His expression could not have been any more neutral.

"I'm not sure what you mean. This doesn't change anything." In a calm and unshaken manner, he headed into the kitchen. "What's for dinner? I'm starving."

"You mean you don't care? Aren't you concerned at all?"

"Jules, did you really think that there was nothing wrong with her? Did you really not know that she was a little person?"

I looked at him, stunned. For the first time I realized that it was not only my friends and family that knew what Taytem was all along, and let us believe otherwise; but it was Colin, too. He had known what she was; that she was never going to the "normal" that I had talked about, and which I had to hold on to.

"She will be fine, Jules. Nothing has changed; she is the same person she always was, and always will be. She will live through this, you will get through this, and she is going to be perfect." He turned toward me, put his arms around me, and pulled me into him. The ability he had to hold me up when my legs would no longer work—that is the memory that will forever be there.

*

That was the first of the changes that would cause my life to rapidly spiral. That was the beginning of the end of the life that at the time seemed so difficult and so tortured. Now it seems so simple, so wonderful—so what I wish I could return to.

*

Colin started becoming very distant. We had taken a couple of trips the summer after Pippa was born, and just shy of her first birthday we had gone on a summer family getaway with his brother and sister-in-law. Colin had insisted that he couldn't take any time off work. That had been his new mantra: make as much money as possible and then retire and enjoy life, and he threw everything he had into it. But that alone couldn't describe the distance I felt—it wasn't just that. He had become moody and withdrawn. He started spending a lot of time in bed or on the couch, even on the weekends, and seemed really kind of disinterested in our family as a whole. Anyhow, he showed up to the trip on Friday night and proceeded to leave early on Sunday, leaving me and the kids behind to stay with the rest of the family. Even while he was there, he was worried, pensive, not himself. Just really irritable: not wanting to spend time together, and being short-tempered when we did. I just assumed that work was weighing him down.

So when I planned another vacation a couple of weeks later (to the same beach-house destination), I told him that he could meet us up on the weekend. This time, though, he insisted that he was going to travel down with me. Colin had had back surgery months before our trip and had never really recovered. He had never taken the time to take care of it. He never attended his physiotherapy, let alone done the exercises they would have told him to do. He'd walked out of the surgery and never looked back. To complicate the matter, he had some degenerative disc disease that would only further irritate his back. I was so worried that he was going to be in a wheelchair at the age of fifty.

The trip was filled with complaints of back pain and stomach issues. As I said, I had sensed a change in Colin, but I just thought it was psychological. Never in my wildest dreams did I think it had some physical dimension. His complaints about his back only made me more resentful. I felt like if he had taken care of his back, gone for the follow-up and rehab, and taken a moment to take care of himself, he would be better by now. The vacation was a miserable week. Colin stayed inside, avoiding us. I was angry that he was avoiding us. It was a constant struggle: me ignoring his overwhelming discomfort, attributing it to psychological issues. I can still remember it like it was yesterday, picturing him in that seventies chair.

In those months prior to Colin's diagnosis, I felt the rift between us growing. We had drifted apart in the past, but it usually only lasted a couple of months, and so I thought this too would go away. During this period, though, every bit of alcohol he drank would go straight to his head, and he would become a belligerent drunk.

One night, we tried to go to a concert. We walked around the stadium for an hour or two before the main act began. We had only had a couple of drinks, and his whole personality began to change. He wasn't himself. Where once we drank to lighten the mood, things had changed. He changed drastically when he drank. He was no longer fun to be around, and it confused me—wondering who this new person was and where it all was coming from. I began to feel regret in the pit of my stomach. I felt so completely and utterly sad. The night that I had planned, the night that I envisioned would bring us back together, would bond us . . . and yet here we were: me, with this man, who was in my company for a total of two hours, and yet was not enjoying our time together so immensely that he had to drink himself into oblivion to just hang out with me. That was the way that I saw it: that he was so miserable in this world, so miserable in the life I had trapped him in—in having another baby, working a job he never truly wanted—that not even for one single night could he stay sober for a small period of time in order for us to enjoy each other.

As we were walking out of the gate, I told him to call the driver. That started a whole process of him calling the limo and talking gibberish, including setting rendezvous points that neither party could feasibly get to. This lasted for a whole hour: on each occasion Colin, who could barely walk, telling me that, this time, he was sure that the driver would be right around the corner. We had walked so far away from the concert venue that, had we gone any further, we might as well have walked all the way home. We got to Lake Shore Drive, and Colin was certain that this was the place. He picked up his phone to call the driver, and told him that he was going to hold up his arms so the limo could see him. He went up on his tiptoes, started waving his arms, and over he tumbled—right into oncoming traffic. Heavy traffic. Dodging cars, he finally hopped up onto the opposite curb, yet now without his cell phone. It had all happened so fast that I hadn't realized he had lost his phone. As angry as I was with him, I was thanking God for not taking his life right there in the middle of Lake Shore Drive. "I lost my phone," was the only thing that he remembered about the terrifying event that had just happened. "Wait, there it is," he said as he darted back out into the busy road, like a squirrel thinking that the risk of death was worth the reward of the acorn.

"Wait, Colin!" I screamed; too late, terrified as the cars came at him and swerved. And then he reemerged: crawling back onto the curb; phone in hand, like he had saved a child from a burning building. I looked at him in disbelief. He had given no wider thought to where he was, or what was happening. All he knew was that he had saved his prized telephone. He shoved the battery back into it, which had fallen on the pavement.

"That's not the right way, Col. Great, you broke the phone. Now we have no way of finding the limo driver. What the hell is wrong with you?! You are a fucking drunk! You have ruined this entire night! I can't believe what you've done; you have ruined it all!" I screamed at him, with such ferocity, such force and anger. The hurt of the evening was stinging me, and I wanted to sting him as well. But I pitied him, standing there. I was confused and hurt, and I was hurt for him. I knew that this evening had meant the same thing to him. I knew he wanted to reconnect. I knew that we had both been happy a few hours before, but it had all gone so wrong so fast. It didn't make any sense. Why did he have to drink so much?

As expected, the next morning brought with it no memories of the night before—only severe vomiting all day and his laying on the couch, miserable. Once again, I was left to clean up the mess of the previous night. I knew then that Colin was not enjoying life. I knew that something was not right. No matter how many bad times we had gone through over the years—and there had been many—we had never gotten to a point where we could not go out, just the two of us, and not have a great time. We'd always end up laughing, forgiving, and getting past whatever the issue was. This time, however, it didn't feel like a simple fix. There was clearly something wrong, something I couldn't put my finger on. Something with him was different... or was it something with me?

For a short while after that night, though, the situation did seem to improve. We spent nights on the porch singing karaoke, hanging out with our friends, and having a good time. Things between us seemed to finally be somewhat better, and we were enjoying one another's company again. In addition, we were starting to plan to the big annual party at our house. Colin and I loved nothing more than to throw big parties, and every year we would have a big Halloween blowout: we'd rent a tent, get four kegs, and everyone—and I do mean everyone—was welcome at our party. This year would be no different.

Colin had been having a hard time at work, losing a lot of money, and had not been feeling well; and the house had all the while been going to seed. I stupidly thought that this big party would be the best way to fix his mood, get the house in order, and have fun. We set the planning in motion, with over two hundred invites going out. By this point, though, Colin's stomach had gotten so incredibly bad that he went to the doctor. The doctor he saw just assumed that he was developing an ulcer. Colin had been given some pretty heavy antacids and then sent on his way.

Nothing seemed to work. In fact, the more antacids he took, the worse his stomach and back pain became. One night, when we were out at dinner, he had a sip of beer and looked as if someone had lit his stomach on fire. He sat in the booth, shifting from side to side, and then excused himself to head to the bathroom. When he returned, he asked me if we could go. I said of course. But on the way home, I lectured him that this was not right. I reasoned that he had been on such heavy-duty antacids that they should have done the trick. There was no way that this was an ulcer.

"This sounds more like a pancreatic problem," I said to him, "like I had after Matthew was born. You need to go back to the doctor, Col, you can't keep ignoring this."

I still felt that something between Colin and I was not right. And, in the period leading up to our party, we grew apart once more. With his obsession with money and getting ahead, Colin had started creating a shield—a preoccupation that I couldn't penetrate. He was changing in ways I couldn't describe, nor fully understand, but I did know that my feelings were hurt. I began to cling to a close friend. I suppose, in a self-preservation way, I was protecting myself from the hurt that I was also feeling. Colin was withdrawn and again barely enjoying our time together. I didn't know what was going on. I thought, at the time, it was jealousy of my friendship with my neighbor. But, looking back, I now see that maybe he had some forethought—maybe he knew that something was about to happen, and he had to pull away from me as well.

*

There are many times in my life I wish I could go back and do things differently, but I can pinpoint that moment as a standout example for when I wish I could have a do-over. I would do things so differently. I wish I had not been so selfish, so caught up in myself. I will probably never be able to forgive myself for not just taking the time to care about what was going on with him, and insist that he go see a doctor.

*

That summer, as I have said, Colin had become inebriated just by looking at alcohol. Indeed, back when he was in college, he would get so drunk that he would get stupid. They used to call it "Barthmode".

Although I had only witnessed it on VERY rare occasions during our fourteen years together, I had begun seeing such changes in him when he would drink. About three drinks in, he would become demanding, silly—but it would then go beyond silly. His personality would change. He would become sloppy and belligerent. He became a different person. "Creepy Colin" was how I termed it. I thought it all stemmed from the stress of his job. I knew that he was putting more risk on his position at work, and I attributed it all to that: the personality changes, the inability to hold his liquor, the preoccupation with making money, clearing debt, paying off the house. He had started taking out life insurance policies: first on himself, and then me.

The Halloween party was now imminent, and Colin was still not feeling better. The couple of recent occasions whereby we had attempted to go out had ended in disaster: Colin either getting way too drunk, else not wanting to drink at all and complaining about excruciating pain in his stomach. A week before the party, Colin finally agreed to go into the hospital, and to stay until they could tell him what was wrong. Truth be told, I think that he just wanted to be able to drink and enjoy the party, and thought the hospital would be able to give him a quick fix.

I remember that I had errands to run that day. "You don't want me to come with you, do you?" I asked.

"No, I'll be fine. You go ahead, and I'll call you when I get back."

*

Likewise, there have been so many times over the years that I have pictured that moment: that last goodbye, and my heading out the door. At that moment in time, I said my last goodbye—not just to Colin, but to my life, my entire world. How many times have I seen someone who lost someone in an accident, a fire, unexpectedly, and they remember that last time: the last time they saw them, the last time they said goodbye. Yet as I headed out the door, I had no idea that I would never again see Colin, my husband, the person he was, again.

*

While I ran errands, preparing for the party, I checked in maybe three or four times, and on each occasion Colin would answer the phone groggily, not knowing anything. I would ask him what they were saying and doing for him. He had no answers whatsoever. By noon, by which point he had been there for four hours, I called one last time.

"What's going on?" I quizzed, almost annoyed.

"Nothing. I don't know what they are doing; they're just running tests."

"Well, what are they saying?"

"They're not saying much of anything. In fact, I haven't seen anyone in a while."

"I am just going to come to the hospital, Colin."

I had this feeling, immediately, that I needed to get there. There was something in my soul that beckoned me, and made me feel it was imperative that I got to that hospital. I began driving erratically: cutting people off, cursing anyone and everyone in my path, trying to go through stoplights. After rally-racing across town I arrived at the hospital, and was quickly ushered into the emergency room where Colin was. He lay on a gurney in front of me: slightly elevated, watching television; and completely unaware that I was standing before him, panting and concerned.

"What's up?" was all that I could muster to say to him. "Have you heard anything yet? Why are you still here?"

He turned to me, completely befuddled.

"The weirdest thing just happened," he said. "The ER doctor came in and said that he'd found something on the ultrasound that he didn't expect to find. And then his pager went off and he rushed out of the room, saying he would be right back."

"When was that?"

"Just a minute ago . . ." he replied, trailing off.

Looking into his eyes, I quickly realized that he had been heavily medicated. Not only was he not complaining of the pain that had plagued him for months, but he seemed without a care in the world.

The doctor came in right at that moment, scanning the room as he did so. He looked at Colin and then at me. A flash of relief came over his face, which instantly changed to pity.

"Are you his wife?" he asked.

"Yes, I am."

"Well, I am very glad you made it."

Made it? For what? Was all I could think. He hadn't even known I was coming.

"As I was saying, Mr. Barth, we saw something on the ultrasound that we hadn't expected to find, so we're all kind of shocked . . ." It was his turn to trail off, and his gaze dropped to the floor. "It appears from the ultrasound that you have a large tumor on the tail of your pancreas. And, in addition, several lesions on your liver. We can't be sure, but we think that it may be cancer. We think that the cancer, which is pancreatic, has metastasized to your liver, but we will need a biopsy to be sure."

Colin and I both sat there. I had heard the doctor, but it was as if I was not listening. For all I understood, he had just told me that Colin had a cold.

"So, what does that mean?" I asked; not really sure that I wanted to hear the answer, and keenly aware that it was not good news.

"That means that we just can't be sure, but it looks like he has several cancerous tumors along his pancreas and liver. I would be very doubtful if these tumors were benign."

I stood there, motionless. I was looking at the doctor, but really looking through him.

Surely he did not say what I think he just said.

But, at the same time, I did know what he was saying.

Colin was in utter shock. I don't know if it was the drugs, or just the sheer surprise of what was being said—probably a combination of the two—but he didn't utter a sound. He didn't question. He didn't cry out. He didn't respond at all. It was like he hadn't heard any of it. We both refused to look at each other. I grabbed his hand and remember squeezing it, although I can't remember if he squeezed back.

"I am really sorry to be giving you this news, Mr. Barth. I have called in a gastro consult. They should be here shortly to take the case and to do your biopsy. I am sorry. I will leave you two alone, but if you have any questions, just call the nurse and she will come get me."

Several hours later, the consult, an Asian woman in her early twenties shuffled in. She was definitely a med student or resident sent in to do the grunt work. She had the social skills of . . . well, none at all. She began to ask Colin questions, and within minutes he was vomiting. After about three questions that went unanswered, she eventually looked up from her clipboard.

"Colin?" she finally asked. "Do you need to take a break?"

"Yes," I snapped, "I think a break would be appropriate since you just told the man he has cancer."

"So, have you been throwing up like this long?" she asked, apparently immediately forgetting that she had just offered to give him a break from the questioning.

"No, he just started throwing up now," I shot back. "Maybe because you told him that he has tumors all over his body!"

Recognizing that Colin was vomiting so profusely, and was so heavily medicated that she was not going to get any real significant answers, she finally finished up her report, and subsequently left the room without hardly uttering another word.

Colin's vomiting lasted well into the evening, eventually subsiding to dry heaving. I really can't remember if we went home, if we spent the night, if we did the biopsy. I can't remember if we called his parents, my parents, who was watching the kids. We left the hospital, having been told they would have the biopsy back on Halloween. We were to meet at a Dr. Petty's office to discuss whatever the results showed.

Looking back, I don't think there was a soul in that room who didn't know what we were looking at and what we were facing—except Colin and I. That said, there was good reason for that. We had been on the receiving end of bad news and poor prognoses before. But also of misdiagnoses. We had been told terrible things by medical professionals that had then never happened. We had worried about awful things that could potentially play out—probably taking years off of our lives in the process—only to be told, forty-eight hours later, that they had been mistaken. So we went home and prayed that we would again be told that things were not what they had initially seemed.

Furthermore, while in the hospital, I had instructed my neighbor to go ahead and cancel our Halloween party. I told her very little, and very briefly, what had happened in the hospital, since I did not really know myself. But, I did tell her the potential of what we were facing.

We were in a small town, and it being that we had invited over two hundred people, the message went out to everyone at once. The parent tree had been alerted, and the rumor mill started to churn—instantly.

That very same day, Jake was playing his last football game. Colin was the head coach, and, true to Colin's spirit, he was going to make it—he had told Jake and the team he would be there, and he was not going to let them down. We left the hospital and headed straight for the field. Colin looked horrible, with no color in his skin, and I knew how incredibly loopy he was from the heavy narcotics. He was still wearing his pajama pants, and a Bears hat covered his head. He popped out of the car almost before I had come to a stop and went to join the other coaches since the game was already in progress. The look of pity on the other parents' faces was too much for me. (Although I had been attempting to hide my shock, and trying to hold onto optimism, I saw everything in their faces.) I hadn't cried up until then; hadn't let it in, or even acknowledged it—but, standing there, seeing the pity in their eyes, it overcame me. One woman noticed my tears and came over, and I began to tell her what the doctors were saying. One of the other mothers then began telling me about her sister-in-law, who had just died from pancreatic cancer, and that her father was a leading specialist in cancer research. God love her, she was trying to be helpful and offer up her services. But it wasn't something I was ready to hear, to accept, or to think about. I tried to give her the signal to stop, but she apparently did not read it correctly, and just continued on.

Out of the corner of my eye I saw Colin confronting the opposing team's coach. He was up in the man's face. I knew in an instant that attending this game had been a bad idea. Colin should have been home in bed. I should have insisted on that, but I felt this was something he needed to do—a promise to Jake that he needed to keep. Suddenly Colin stopped yelling, turned around, and headed off the field. I gathered the kids as Colin hopped into my mother's car, saying he would meet me at home. We were just a mile from the house, yet by the time me and the kids made it back, he was already up in bed and fast asleep.

We had forty-eight hours at home—none of which I remember, besides trying desperately to keep the kids away from Colin. I mistakenly and very naively thought that a little rest and relaxation could somehow cure the deadliest form of cancer there was.

We had scheduled an appointment to consult with the oncologist, Dr. Petty. We showed up right on time: numb, and in shock. I can relive the physical movements we made to get there, but none of the thought processes.

As we stood in the room, Colin began to pace. I don't think he and I'd had a conversation beyond "Do you need anything?" since we had returned home from the hospital, but as he strode around that room with fervor, he spoke out.

"This is nothing, Jules," he expounded, very confidently. "Really, this is nothing; everything is fine. But I get it—this is a wake-up call. I need to really start taking better care of myself. When we leave here, when this is over, I am going to start working out and taking care of myself. This is a wake-up call."

For the first time in forty-eight hours, I exhaled, my teeth unclenched, and I felt some oxygen enter my body. Yes, of course they were wrong! What sad, sick, sadistic fate would bring this down on two people who had suffered so much together already? This couldn't really be happening. He was so right: it was all right there in front of me. This was a wake-up call. We looked at each other as if to say, "Whew . . . thank God that's over". We were both so positive that it wouldn't, couldn't, *shouldn't*, be us again, that we reconnected, sitting in that room as we waited for the doctor to walk in and say, "Yes, guys, false alarm. Now be warned, you aren't getting any younger. Go home, work out, eat better, go on vacation for Christ's sake; you deserve some time alone, the two of you". And we would walk out, hand-in-hand, repaired, ready to rebuild and start anew.

The door opened and Dr. Petty walked in. I almost felt like I should have one hand on the door in preparation for saying, "Thanks so much; we'll be back in a year for a physical or something".

"Your father and stepmom are in the waiting room," said the doctor. "Do you mind if they come in too?"

"Sure, why not?"

Colin was so carefree—more so than I had seen him in months. His mind had eased and his fear was gone. He was somewhere on vacation, even now as we spoke: his mind had gone ahead, awaiting the arrival of his body.

His father and stepmom shuffled into the room and quickly took their seats.

Dr. Petty took a seat in front of me and looked at Colin. Colin was ready for the good news to roll off the doctor's tongue. Colin gave him a nod, almost like he was saying, "Nope, I'm good. You go on without me; I already heard this part".

"The results showed exactly what we assumed they would," he began.

Colin and I both looked at him with grins on our faces, completely not hearing what he was saying. In our minds we had both resolved to entertaining our colluded scenario as long as we could.

"The cancer, which started in the pancreas, has metastasized to your liver, and you're not eligible for surgery. It's the worst-case scenario."

I'm sure Colin heard him physically, but he continued to pace like he had not heard him mentally.

"Well, what are our options?" Colin asked, as if snapping out of a trance.

"Well, there really aren't any. There are really no drugs that have shown much efficacy with pancreatic cancer—especially cancer that is this far advanced. You can try Gemcitabine; it is the only chemo drug that is approved for this kind of cancer. But I have to be honest with you—won't be cured. There is no cure for what you have."

Colin looked at him incredulously and headed for the door.

At that point, Dr. Petty knelt by me and whispered in a low voice, apparently intended for keeping the others in the room from hearing:

"He has a very limited time. Probably a couple of weeks at best. Don't waste your time chasing cures; it will only make him sicker and will prove nothing. Take him home now and enjoy whatever time he has left here with his kids."

With those last words of what I guess he thought was tough love, he stood up and left the room, leaving me behind with my jaw resting on the floor.

Tears wouldn't come, they didn't even want to be present at this. I was in shock, the kind of shock where you think there must be some mistake, and in an instant there was flash-pan anger. I had totally forgotten that Diana and Ben were in the room, and I got up, didn't say a word to them and started heading out the door. I was muttering under my breath, "Take him home and let him die my ass . . . that is what they said to his mom . . . really, this is the best you can do? Way to support us, to find us help, that is . . . What kind of a shit doctor doesn't even try to help . . . he is *thirty-five*." And then my muttered words became louder. I wanted them to hear me; I wanted them to hear my anger at their throwing in the towel before the fight had begun. Obviously they had no idea who Colin was, what his genetics had shown through his mother. They had told her she wouldn't make it through the initial surgery, and then given her weeks, and here we were eighteen years later; twenty-three grandchildren whom she would never have met. That is what we were going to do to . . . we had saved Taytem, we had taken a girl who they told us would never walk, would never talk, would be nothing but a vegetable, and that "vegetable" was at kindergarten right as we were standing in that office. They were wrong, just as all of those other experts had been along the road in our lives. "They dont't know we are Barths. They don't know that we don't go down with the ship: we scratch, we claw, we fight, and we survive . . . He is thirty-five, really? No advice, nothing? He has four kids, for God's sake!" My voice had begun to become loud and belligerent. "That's it, huh?! 'Go home and die'?! You are wrong. You are wrong. He is going to survive this, we are going to prove you wrong."

I stormed out into the waiting room—the same waiting room that fifteen minutes earlier had held so much promise—and realized that, as I was making my grand exit, I had forgotten about finding Colin. Seconds later, he came through the door, totally drugged up and completely unfazed. Yes, he was a little peaked, but for someone who had just been given a death sentence he was completely composed; completely anger-free, worry-free. He was ready to go home and begin the fight of his life. I often thank God that he had not heard what Dr. Petty had said to me.

We got into the car. and I was in complete shock. The kind of shock where you don't know what you are feeling, or if you are even alive. I sat down first and Colin inched his way into the car. For a brief moment, I forgot; I forgot what we were just told. I looked at him and, in a flash, I just saw Colin: not the dying Colin, the pained Colin, just Colin. I was quickly shaken back to reality when the wincing began and he guided his leg into the car slowly. "Hey Col, do I have room on that side?" He turned to look to his right, or at least I thought he did. "Yeah, you are clear," he said. I began to pull out and heard metal against metal. Colin didn't flinch, he didn't even notice, he just looked straight ahead. I had another moment of flash-pan anger—"You just said that . . ."—but soon trailed off when I realized that not only was he not even present in his own body, but how stupid of me to ask someone who was just told they are going to die of cancer and who is drugged out of their ever-loving mind, to gauge whether I have room to back out of a parking space. I left the scene of that crime: not intentionally, I am not sure that it even registered that someone else's car was involved at all. I didn't until months later even recall the event, when I went to get in the car and looked down to see that there was a dent in the passenger side. I had shuttered quickly as the events of that day flooded back, and felt instant remorse at not leaving a note or acknowledging that someone else was involved. As I say, I was in utter shock. The mind has a miraculous way to blocking out things. When stress becomes too great, the mind can just shut off, protect us, allow us to continue on.

The ride home was silent. I was in denial over the information and, true to my nature, was devising a plan. First I would call the MD Anderson Cancer Center. Then I would get online. And then, as I had some very wealthy people in high places, I would call in all the favors I could. We would travel, we would find the experts, he would be fine. He was going to live to watch Pippa walk down the aisle. Like his mother: the oldest surviving ovarian cancer patient then in the US, who would meet all twenty-three of her grandchildren, living on for over twenty years on borrowed time The fight was on, a challenge was being waged—one I was strong enough for, and ready to fight.

With all the boys' birthdays being in November (Jake's and Matthew's birthdays are a day apart, and Colin's followed at the end of the month), October and November had always seen our house full of parties and celebrations. Desperately needing a distraction, and needing to be surrounded by people for an occasion that was not "like a wake" at our home, I decided that we should have a combined birthday party for them. I needed to have people in the house again: the kind of company who would come to our home with emotions other than fear, sadness, or pity. I thereby invited a very small group of family and our closest friends.

They were all eager to help, and refused to let me cook (or in fact do anything). They came for a potluck, and for just one night Colin came down in his favorite sweater, with a genuine smile on his face, happy to see everyone. He had drugged himself up enough to join the human race, which was always a tricky cocktail. For the first time, we could all forget—if only for a moment—what we were facing. Colin stood taller than I had seen him in months. He was cordial and lighthearted, being surrounded by his lifelong and family friends. He was calmer than I had seen in a long time, too, and willing to be part of this world for just this moment. We all had dinner, and Colin stayed for about an hour, opening gifts and enjoying himself, before he had to excuse himself to disappear once again to the vacant upstairs room that had become his shelter.

I had gotten to work very quickly on finding somewhere that could offer a cure. I inquired about the experimental drugs I learned of, and contacted specialists who could in theory take out his organs and do a 3-D operation of his pancreas. (Sure, it would take seventy-two hours for the operation, but they might be able to do it.) And then I found a doctor who was experimenting with some new cancer drug, and decided this was it: this was our cure. I sent that doctor an email, pleading with him to just consider taking Colin—only to find out that he was not the figure running the study. It was being done at another center, and we could be put on a waiting list (we had missed it by a month). I contacted them as well: begging them, crying, only to have it confirmed that there was no space available.

Although I was not facing the facts, Colin's body was; and I quickly began to see that my medical search, my insistence that we needed to travel far and wide to find the wizard, not only was not going to happen, but that I was wasting precious time we didn't have.

At the very beginning of our journey, right when Colin found out what we were facing, his mother—herself having connections, after battling ovarian cancer for at that point twenty plus years—had conducted her own research and found that one of the leading specialists was located at the University of Chicago, which was literally only about an hour from our home. We went to see the woman in question, but there was something about her that just didn't seem to ring true. She said all the right things, paused at all the right times to exhibit sympathy for the young husband and father of four, but I didn't believe that she really meant it—I didn't believe that she really cared. After trudging downtown to see her, and waiting for hours, we got nothing more than "Sorry, I have a study, but it is closed". *Come again soon, or don't.* Colin was a lot kinder than I was (possibly because he was more drugged, or resigned to accept his fate), but I could have decked her. I walked out of that room seething with anger. After wasting our time, that was all she had to offer.

Around the same time, I had finally scored an appointment with the foremost specialist of pancreatic cancer at the leading cancer hospital in Dallas, MD Anderson. The only problem was that he had been on vacation. I had faxed over all the information, secured the appointment for right when he returned, and I suppose that date was the decision deadline I was giving myself for figuring out what to do.

I was running on fumes. I was trying to deal with the kids; simultaneously avoiding and taking care of Colin; researching a doctor; and freaking out that we didn't have money to pay the mortgage.

You see, Colin *had* had plenty of life insurance. He had taken out a million-dollar policy two years before his diagnosis. I thought at the time that it was a waste: *What thirty-three-year-old needs a million-dollar policy?!* But it was post- 9/11, and since he worked downtown I think that had sent him to invest in it.

However, back on that fateful day when we were driving from Dr. Petty's office—the very day he was told that he was going to die—he said but one thing on the way home:

"I am so sorry, Jules, I'm so sorry. I forgot to pay the life insurance three months ago. I totally just stopped paying."

At the time, for me to acknowledge this admission would ruin me for two reasons. One, I refused to believe that I would need life insurance for him, because he was NOT going to die; and two, I was angered by his making such a silly oversight. But . . . for me to be mad that a dying man had forgotten to pay the life insurance policy? Well, what a horrible, miserable human being would I be to acknowledge that, and to make him feel worse. I had therefore said nothing in the car other than, "Who cares, Colin? You can't think about that right now; it doesn't matter", and that too had been right before he drifted off to sleep: hopefully knowing that I loved him more than life itself, and certainly more than life insurance. I cared about *him*, not about what would happen in a life without him.

But in those weeks after the diagnosis, I started to realize that *I was scared to death*. I couldn't afford four kids—I hadn't worked in ten years; and even when I *did* work, I sucked at it! Colin had made a lot of money over the year leading up to this event, but he had lost it all—over $500,000. Those months where we drifted apart and his entire personality had changed were bad ones in the economy. Whether it was the illness and not feeling well, or just things that would have happened anyway, he had lost nearly all of his trading profits and our savings. It was all gone—and so there was no life insurance, no money in the bank, no husband, and four kids.

I was crazy on fire. I would spend all day trying to get him into a clinical trial, trying to get him a cure, and all night listing and shipping things on eBay to pay the bills. Any other spare moments were spent taking care of the kids. But in all that time, Colin was left to fend for himself: not only emotionally, but physically. I would come upstairs, bring him his medications, and then return to whatever other hat I was wearing at the time. I was terrified of losing the house, losing him, losing it all. My life had disappeared in the time it took to take one ultrasound; the life that I thought was so difficult had become a breeze. It had become the dream life that I would no longer have.

On the Friday afternoon at the end of the three weeks—just as I was getting ready for Dallas, knowing I had to order tickets online in the next day or two—we got a call back from the leading Chicago specialist we had gone to see, Dr. Helen Kinler. She had been the very first specialist we had visited, who had had very little to lend to the conversation, and I had been put off by her lack of empathy or solutions. Though I was now beginning to understand that perhaps that wasn't about the specialist's personality; maybe it is what they had to do to protect themselves. Colin, my loved one, was dying of cancer, and Helen and other doctors like her would have met many strangers who then became people they cared about, families they got to know, that didn't survive. There had to be some part of them that developed a thick skin, otherwise I don't know how they could remain objective and do their job; find a cure. Whereas once I thought doctors must go into it with that type of outlook, I had now been in the medical "world" long enough to know that if you truly want to make a difference and help, you have to be on the outside. The inner track will probably eat you alive.

We were informed that she now did have an opening on her trial (I didn't even want to know why), meaning there was a space for Colin. Knowing that we were going to MD Anderson the following Tuesday, I was so torn. *Do I wait it out, and lose the spot at MD Anderson? Or do I take this experimental spot at the University of Chicago?*

Colin was becoming sicker. In fact, I had taken him down for one last consult at Northwestern Hospital the week before, and he had been so out of his mind with pain that he had been unable to sit at all the entire time we were there. He had paced like a caged animal, only to find out that the doctor we met with—who was probably one of the kindest specialists we had seen up until that point—had nothing of any value to offer him.

And so when they called that Friday, I asked Lauren, Helen's assistant, "Well, do we have to let you know right now, right this minute?" and she definitively said that I did.

It was the hardest decision I have ever made, and probably the one I will question for the rest of my days on this earth.

"Okay, then yes, we will be in the study."

Lauren told me that she would secure his position. Yet, after hanging up, I quickly went to work devising a backup plan. I called

MD Anderson to ask them what they thought. If it didn't work out, could we still come? I didn't want to screw up all the work I had done getting him to the country's leading specialist. I dialed the contact that I had at MD Anderson. I got Lisa on the phone and I began to explain.

"My husband Colin has been waiting for an appointment with Dr. Smith because he was on vacation for two weeks . . . and we have been accepted into a study with Helen Kinler at the University of Chicago . . ." I was telling the story so quickly, not pausing even to take a breath. ". . . I just want to make sure that if we decide to take a position in this study, that we will still be able to come see you. If by chance he does really well and we can move on to more aggressive treatment, or if he doesn't do so well, can we still come to MD Anderson? I need to know that if I make this decision that I am not closing any doors. I am just so afraid that right now he is not well enough to travel and that we have this opportunity available right here, but I don't want to miss the opportunity for him to be seen by the best . . .

". . . Thank you, thank you so much. That is exactly what I needed to hear."

She had said that our best bet would be to give the University of Chicago study a try. I cancelled the MD Anderson appointment, called my mother, cried, worried that I was making the wrong decision, and tried to believe that the fates were finally giving us a break and this could be it.

We were supposed to go down on the Monday to sign the paperwork to begin the study. But, later that Friday, around three p.m., Lauren called me back, telling me that she had made a mistake. She could not hold the spot until Colin physically came downtown and signed all the paperwork.

"Well, can we just wait until Monday? How many people are waiting on this spot?" I questioned.

She seemed very insistent that we came immediately. There were only ninety people in the study, and I would guess hundreds wanted in. I think that Colin must have been catapulted to the top of the list because of his age and his family history of beating cancer. If there was a genetic link between treatment success and this cancer, Colin would prove to be a goldmine for Helen.

"So we need to come right now, tonight?" I asked her in disbelief. For anyone who has ever been or lived in Chicago, the prospects of making it all the way from the north side to the south side on a Friday afternoon would take a miracle in its own right.

I had been out with my mother when Lauren had called to tell me. I hung up the phone and broke into tears. We had been out together for no more than an hour, having just dropped Matthew off at preschool, and after that talking about which decision was best for Colin. I feverishly started dialing the phone. I knew that if there was ONE person in the world who could be objective, who would put Colin first, who would be able to put everyone else aside to see what was best for Colin—and it was his mother. After many rings, Diana picked up the phone. Without hesitation I quickly explained the situation.

"I need your help, Diana," I said, having given the overview, "I don't know what to do. I want to make sure that I am doing the right thing, that I am making the right decision for Colin . . ."

"Julie, I think Colin would be better suited staying here, don't you?" was her only reply, with no other questions to ask. "I think that if you feel like that is the right decision, then I agree; I stand behind it one hundred percent."

"Okay, thanks, Diana. I will keep you posted." I hung up the phone and looked to my mother.

"I need to go home and get Colin to take him downtown, right now. If I don't they could give the study space to someone else," before adding, "He is so sick Mom, am I doing the right thing dragging him downtown right now? He is at home, throwing up: how am I going to get him in a car to drive through traffic? What do I do?!"

My mother looked me squarely in the eye.

"Julie, if you are afraid that you are not going to be able to get him to downtown Chicago, forty-five minutes from home in traffic, how on earth do you think you are going to get him across the country? God is giving you a sign, an opportunity here, you have to take it."

"Will you watch the kids?"

"Of course I will. Just go home, get him, and get the papers signed. You can always still go to MD Anderson."

I raced home and up the stairs. I found Colin half sitting, his head propped up, glasses still on. It was cold and gloomy outside, and the window shades were all drawn; the room was completely dark.

"Col?" I whispered, as I inched toward him. No answer. "Col?" He moved his head slightly and looked at me out of the corner of his eye. "Col, we have to go downtown."

"Downtown? Why do we have to go downtown?" he asked, incredulous.

"We have to go down and sign some papers. They have a space available downtown in that study with Dr. Kinler—just one space available. But we have to go down and sign the papers tonight, or someone else will get the space."

He looked from me to the television and then back at me. Propelling himself from the bed, he started a mad race toward the bathroom and all I heard for the next ten minutes was retching. The guilt welled up inside me. *If I had only let him sleep* . . . I had disturbed the very few hours in which he had found any peace in the past couple of weeks.

"Col, I am so sorry." I walked this conversation cautiously, for at that very moment I was beginning to doubt my own decision. Looking at him, at his misery, how could I ask him to right now hop into a car and be driven for hours on end. It was a Friday afternoon in Chicago. Traffic was always bad on a Friday, from the northside to the end of the southside—that forty-five minutes could quickly and easily become four hours, and frequently did. "Col, we have to go, we have to go now."

When he replied his eyes had already closed again. "Can't they fax it or something? Can't we do this Monday? I don't understand." He started to become less agitated, and more childlike: pleading with me; trying to understand why on earth I would be asking this of him right now.

"If someone signs it before you do, then you won't get the space."

"But I thought we were going to MD Anderson?"

"Col, please, come on, all you have to do is get up and into the car, I promise. We will get there, all you have to do is sign, and then we will come right back home."

I began running around the room, getting his clothes, his socks, putting his "to go" stuff together.

I pulled out of the driveway the way that I always did, but realized that even the motion of backing up and the knee-jerk movements that were part of driving were not going to go down well. I was going to have to take it slowly. It reminded me of when I broke my arm as a child—in that, for Colin, every single movement of the car was excruciating.

We headed downtown and, sure enough, we were stuck in traffic for over an hour and a half. It was Friday rush hour, and although I knew it would be horrible, I had no idea how bad it actually could be. For the entire drive, Colin sat stone-faced, looking ahead, moaning every once in a while. He would lean forward and cry and plead with me, and then look at me angrily, as if to say "Why are we doing this again? Why are you torturing me?"

We got there, and within minutes were escorted to a waiting room. Lauren was pretty and unassuming; very young, too, and not tainted by years of watching people die (her innocence was still intact; you could see it in her face). She had blonde hair pulled back in a ponytail, wore khaki pants and a white coat, and although she was trying hard to be at ease, Colin's very apparent misery was something she was not prepared for. She kept trying to talk to him, yet received no answers in return. As she explained exactly what the study entailed, the specifics, the start time, he refused to look at her; he refused to look at anything but the ground. I knew well enough that he was not even present.

Lauren told us that Colin was going to need to come down and repeat the scans and blood work, and that the chemo side effects were very minimal. Most people experienced at worst a little nausea, but compared to the shape he was presently in it would likely not do anything—in fact, it would probably make him feel *better*. Colin signed on the line, and when he was finished he excused himself to go to the bathroom. When he left the room, Lauren leaned in and confessed something that I believe might have been the final gift that the fates gave to me—a conciliatory recognition that perhaps I might have made the right decision that day.

"You know, I am so glad that I called you back and had you come down. When I found out that there was only one space available, and that you were not guaranteed it until you officially signed the papers, I began to get worried. I got a call right before you came in that there was a woman in San Francisco who signed the papers at exactly 4:13."

I looked down at my watch to see that it was 5:09, and Colin had only just now signed it.

"So we didn't get in?!" I snapped. "I don't understand?"

"No, since you all were so close, for ethical reasons they have agreed to take you both. We had to go to bat for you, but now you are both in."

I never told Colin about the circumstances of that day: that we had been beaten out, that someone had beat us in the signature; or how lucky it was that we made it into the study when we did.

As we sat in traffic on the way home, you could see all the way ahead for miles. The night had come, and the glare from the lights of the trucks, and the street lights, and from the cars in general, all around us, was more excruciating to Colin's head than the sun had been. But when he closed his eyes it became even worse—like when you have had too much to drink, and the spinning brought on when you shut your eyes then makes the nausea kick up a notch further. We sat in that car: him wrenching, moaning, crying, for another two hours on the ride home, me all the while helpless to improve his situation. I tried to reach for him several times, to rub his arm, to hold his hand and to run my finger through his sweat-soaked hair, as he writhed in pain.

The next morning, we were due downtown again in order to run through all the testing. I had called Colin's stepfather Ben to take him. Colin was having a somewhat better day, and since it was a Saturday and not during rush hour, the trip took them a third of the time and they were home quickly. Colin came back and acknowledged everyone. I think just the prospect of beginning something had lifted his spirits just enough to let him join this world for a short period of time.

He went up to bed, but within a couple of hours came back down, complaining that he was having a hard time breathing. Off we headed to the emergency room. Within an hour of being there (the sad irony of being terminally ill is that they get you in right away; apparently dying catapults you to the front of the line), we were told that Colin had two huge pulmonary embolisms in his chest, which were preventing him from breathing, and although all of the back pain that he was experiencing had appeared to be tumor-related, it was in fact down to the restriction from the blood clots. He was a ticking time bomb. Those embolisms could have been dislodged at any time, and traveled to his heart—but they had stayed put: just long enough to add more torture to his world. He was hospitalized and put on heavy-duty blood thinners to try and get the clots to dissipate.

About a day into it, he started developing this nasty rash from head to toe. It looked like someone had beaten him all over. However, although it looked uncomfortable and miserable, he barely seemed to notice. The doctors came in to inform us that he was days away from dying, had he not come in. I am not sure why they shared that information—to tell us of his "luck"? Or to warn us to not ignore symptoms any longer?—but, in any event, it didn't seem lucky at all.

At the end of that night, I hopped in the car to head home, my head pounding. Literally pounding. It was raining, so the glare from the headlights were shining brightly into my eyes and the strong lamps of the street lights were reflecting off of those. It was hard to see, and I had forgotten my glasses. It would take no more than fifteen minutes to get home, and I was anxious to get some sleep and peel off this day and get under the covers, but as I drove along I saw a detour ahead of me, which led me onto a path that, although living here for over . . . well, all my life . . . I had no idea where it was going. I finally admitted it to myself, on that ride home: I was lost. I was lost, and stuck, and had no one, no one to help me home.

No one else would ever be Colin, and the person I thought I was—so confident, so independent—wanted nothing more than to turn back the hands of the clock and have him back. Not the man that he had become, the person in so much pain. My Colin: the love of my life, my world; who could make me smile, laugh, and make everything okay. I realized, on that drive home—rain pounding my car, driving along lost—that I wouldn't have my world back ever again. It was gone, and I never realized how much I needed Colin; how much I needed him to be there with me, guiding me home.

His rash continued for days, and so did the blood thinners. At this point, I was taking him to the doctor on a daily basis. He needed to have his blood measured, but my major concern was the pain. He was taking the highest dosage of all the painkillers he could have, but if he wasn't sleeping then he was pacing. He would pace from one end of our room to the next, sit in our antique rocking chair, rock for a few minutes, and then get up again to pace the floor. From the very moment this all began—from the minute he found out that he had cancer—he developed this leg shake. He would take his feet and rub them together over and again, just shake and rub, and this would go on continually. It almost appeared that he was continually trying to shake the pain from his very soul out through his feet.

When I would walk over to him, I always put my hands on his feet in an effort to calm him and stop his feet from the perpetual movement. He would always look up at me, astonished that I had touched him. He had no awareness of his constant movement—it was completely and utterly involuntary.

We went to the oncologist the day after returning home, to try to get his thinning levels under control. We walked in to have his blood levels taken by my "favorite" doctor—the one who told me to take him home and let my four young children watch him die without even trying to fight it. Colin, again pacing, had his blood test done and was ready to go home, but I wouldn't just go. I was not going to leave there until they gave him something to make the pain more manageable. Colin kept looking to me, pleading with me to just take him home and let him hop back into bed, shut out the world again, to pull the covers up over his head and try to just exist.

The doctor was no longer there, and apparently no one thought Colin's pain was worthy of "bothering" him on his day off. Finally, the nurse realized that although everyone around me was telling me to pick myself up and take Colin home to suffer, that I was not going until someone listened. She got on the phone and within five minutes had a script for a stronger painkiller: one I hoped would provide a modicum of relief. Little did I know that they were right—relief was not to be found for Colin. The mental anguish and the physical pain of what he was facing and what the cancer was doing to his body was never to ease. That is the part that will never leave me, that feeling of helplessness. The guilt of watching it all: the pain, the pacing, the crying, the vomiting; watching it from the sidelines. I was okay, standing there on the outside, watching him plead with the world to let him have a day of peace, a day of no pain, and I could do nothing to help, nothing but perpetually ask him "are you alright?" when I knew the answer was "no".

I started to become more vacant: my personality leaving my body a little more each day, becoming more and more disconnected. I started avoiding him. My anger grew at having to watch it and live through it. I became preoccupied with stupid things: money, fundraising, the kids' college funds, the mortgage—things that didn't matter, yet which could distract me from what was really going on: distract me from watching the person I loved more than anyone in the world suffer so intensely; and distract myself from not being able to do anything for him. He began therapy with a chiropractor I knew from high school. The treatments were expensive, but I told him I didn't care.

Colin's tests had all been done at the University of Chicago, where he was signed up for the study and ready to begin. We were both extremely optimistic and eagerly awaiting the treatment. The weeks beforehand had brought out probably some of our best parenting—and the worst. At times when I was too overwhelmed, I would spend the day immersed in them: finding joy in watching them carry on with life, no matter what was going on with Colin. Each day they were just living, like kids do, oblivious; and there were days I was able to join them in that venture. However, when Colin needed a ride or was having a particularly bad day, they were left to their own devices.

Colin was scheduled for chemo starting Monday morning, very early, but, the Friday before, Pippa—now thirteen months old—had developed a fever with vomiting. She had spent the two previous nights waking up in the middle of the night, vomiting, and then going back to sleep; then waking in the morning, not acting right, yet displaying no "real", visible signs of illness. (Or maybe I was too overwhelmed to see them.) By Saturday night Pippa had a raging fever of one hundred and five, and was vomiting and non-responsive. Knowing the importance the first day of chemo would bring, and wanting so badly to be there with Colin and to hold his hand, I was in a quandary as to what I should do. Colin was not well enough to even get out of bed without assistance, much less get food or take care of himself, but I had this little soul who also needed her mother. I went to Colin and tried to explain the situation to him.

"Colin, Pippa is really, really sick. I think I should take her to the ER. I am afraid she has something like meningitis—but I know you are starting chemo tomorrow. I don't know what to do. I need you to tell me what to do."

He barely glanced up at me. I started weighing the options. I knew in my heart that if it were me laying there sick, or if Colin had been well enough to make any decisions, he would most definitely tell me to go with Pippa. Although he was sick, I felt—again in my heart—that he could take care of himself, or find the right people around him to help out. So I tried a different line of questioning.

"Colin, Colin . . ." I shook him softly. He looked up at me, half-aware, with no recollection of the brief conversation from a moment before. "I have to take Pippa to the ER. I can't go with you in the morning. Who do you want me to call to take you? Who do you want to take you to chemo tomorrow?"

"Anyone but my mother. I just can't handle it—anyone but my mom or Ben."

Since Colin had been diagnosed, for the first time *he* was the one having a problem with his mother. When we had gone to the doctor's office to get the results, his mother was doing some sort of "commercial" out of town. I still have no idea where or when that came about—I didn't care enough at the time to listen to any of the details—but I think it hurt Colin tremendously. After all those years of Colin standing at his mother's side, worrying about her cancer and her illnesses, and at a time when he was sick and needed his mom, she left town. I think it felt like shades of his father's leaving him. So I was stuck. The one person who I could think of calling was his best friend, Kevin. Kevin and Col had known each other since middle school. I knew that it was going to be a long, trying day. Kevin was the one person I knew could sit at Col's side and not feel the need to engage, to make idle chitchat. Kevin was a lawyer who had graduated from Madison and quickly went to work with the public defender in Milwaukee on some pretty indigent cases. His wife Savannah was now pregnant, and they had moved back to Evanston so I picked up the phone in a panic and called him.

"Kevin, it's Julie . . . Pippa is really, really sick and I have to go to the hospital l with her . . . I don't have anyone who can take him. It's early in the morning, so I totally understand if you can't do it. I just need someone to take him down; it's an all-day event at the University of—"

He stopped me mid-sentence. "What time? I will be there."

I gave him as many specifics as I could. He would be at our house at six a.m. to head downtown and check in, and they would tell him what to do from there.

I hung up the phone and went over to Colin.

"Kevin is going to take you downtown to chemo, Col, is that alright?" He nodded, eyes closed. "And I'm going to take Pippa to the hospital. My mom is on her way."

Again, a nod; not a nod of caring or understanding—just a nod of "can you leave me alone now?".

I picked Pippa up from her crib and waited by the door for my mother. When I saw the headlights of her car, I headed out, waving to her as I passed in my rush to the hospital.

After waiting all night in the emergency room with Pippa, who by this time was dehydrated, non-responsive, and receiving fluids, we were finally given a room. My heart was so heavy: thinking about

Colin, worrying whether Kevin came to get him, whether they got to the appointment on time—whether Colin had even been able to get out of bed and make the trip.

Just prior to Colin's getting sick, he had gotten the new iPhone right after it was released. I didn't understand his annoying infatuation with the phone, but it quickly became his window to the outside world. And so what at first had seemed like the scourge of our lives ended up often being the only way that we could communicate. I spent the day texting him several times, and he would answer me with one word every so often, which was enough to let me know that he was still out there.

It was determined that Pippa had a kidney infection (she'd had a bladder infection that went on so long it had backed up into her kidneys). As much as I needed to go home, to go to Colin, I kept looking at Pippa's face. She was so terrified. Unlike me, she had never been in a hospital. I had spent so many days, weeks, months in hospitals for the previous six years that there were parts of me that hated the very sight of them—and other parts of me that felt oddly at home. Nothing that they took out or came at her with, nothing in that room, was foreign to me. I knew what everything was for and how to operate every piece of machinery. But Pippa had no idea where she was, what she was doing there, or how she would ever get out.

As the day stretched into the evening, Colin stopped texting me back. I had also kept in touch with Kevin, messaging him to get his thoughts on the whole situation. Finally, at seven p.m., I got the call from Kevin that he had just dropped Colin home, safe and sound. He had found Colin's mother there, sitting in my room, and had put Colin off to bed. Although it had been a very long day for Colin, he had done well, made it through round one, and was now in bed asleep as far as Kevin knew.

"I'm going to head back to Madison now," Kevin told me.

"Madison? Why are you going to Madison?" I asked, knowing that at the time his wife Sarah was over seven months pregnant.

"I am just heading home."

It didn't dawn on me until that very minute that, although he had talked of moving to Evanston, Kevin had not actually made the move back yet. He had gotten the call from me the night before—in Madison, four hours from Chicago—that Colin needed a ride to the city forty-five minutes from us, and instead of asking me why I was calling him, or whether there was someone closer to give him a ride, or even asking if I had a clue that Kevin was so far away, he said nothing but, "Sure, what time?" He had gotten in the car, left his extremely pregnant wife, and driven four hours. Without hesitation. He had done that for Colin without even batting an eye.

"Julie..."

Diana was on the other end of the phone: audibly shaken, upset, and quite possibly pissed.

"Julie, Colin just got home and he is so sick I don't know what to do. Kevin came here, just dropped him off and gave me no information. He just dropped him off and he is non-responsive, he isn't answering my questions."

I was completely taken back. I had just gotten off of the phone with Kevin not more than ten minutes earlier, who had made it sound as if the day went fine. Colin was safely tucked into bed, he had seen Diana, the whole thing was alright. There had been no indication in Kevin's conversation that anything out of the ordinary, anything that wasn't supposed to happen, happened, so I was caught entirely off guard.

"I don't understand Diana, I just talked to Kevin and he said everything was alright."

"Well, all I know is that Colin is not answering any of my questions."

"I will call Kevin right now and ask him if he knows what time he is supposed to be there tomorrow."

I hung up the phone—the kind of hang up that you think can shatter the earpiece on the phone itself. I then grabbed it again and called Kevin back.

"Hi Kevin, I am really sorry to bother you . . . Diana just called me and said that you dropped Col off without giving her any instructions, just dropped him off and took off quickly, and now she is concerned about anything she is supposed to do, when he is supposed to be back tomorrow . . ."

"Julie . . ." his voice sounded like I had hit him; like I had wounded him in some way. ". . . Julie, I talked to Diana, I told her what they told me, I had a ten-minute conversation with her, I gave her the paperwork . . . I don't have any other information, I am really sorry . . ."

At that point I instantly wished that I had not called Kevin back, thereby pulling him into this cry for attention from my mother-in-law, this need to make it all about her.

"I know Kevin. I am so sorry I called you, I know you did."

I hung up the phone and began feverishly calling the University of Chicago. I knew that phoning Diana back, confronting her, and telling her how I felt would be fruitless for everyone. So instead I started dialing each of my (very limited) contacts in order to find out what time Colin was supposed to be back there.

"Diana, it's Julie," came my voice not long after. "I just called around downtown and they don't know what time to have Colin there, so I am going to call back first thing in the morning to get the information for you. I will make sure to wake up early and stat calling and let you know. Are you there alone, is Colin okay?"

"He is sleeping, but very sick and non-responsive. Ben is going to stay here with me tonight."

I awoke with a start at the hospital as the CMT came in to take Pippa's vitals. The fever had finally broken, but as I snatched up my watch I panicked. It was six-thirty a.m., and I had to find out what time Colin was due back downtown. By seven I finally managed to get someone on the phone, who told me that Colin should head downtown early, as early as possible in fact, because he was supposed to have blood work done. I called the house and, when no one answered, then continued to do so every half-hour. This carried on until *noon*. Come one p.m., I was frantic. I was trapped, unable to breathe, having a panic attack. All I knew was that the last time that I heard from Diana, at nine p.m. the night before, Colin was non-responsive and throwing up. By two p.m., my mother had dropped the kids off at the house after school with a babysitter and come to the hospital to keep me company. She walked into the door to find me in tears, shaking, pacing, out of my mind with worry; convinced that surely Colin was dead, or on the verge of death—there was no other explanation. At half two, after hours of crying, I exhaustedly tried Ben's cell phone one more time.

"Hello?" he answered, without a hint of urgency in his voice.

"Ben, what's going on? Is Colin alright?"

"Nothing; we just walked in the door," was his reply.

I began to tremble with anger, realizing at that very moment that the silence, although construed as unintentional, was my punishment for not including Diana the previous day.

"We just got back from downtown."

"Why didn't you call me? I thought Colin was dead . . ." Tears streamed down my face, my teeth were gritted, my hands clenched involuntarily. "I thought he was *dead*, Ben! I have been trying to call for hours! How could you do that?"

Unable to speak further, I hung up the phone.

The next time the phone rang, it was Colin, apologizing for not being there to answer my call himself. He told me that he was so sick that he hadn't charged his iPhone the night before, and he didn't know that I was worried or that I didn't know where he was. His voice was so faint and sick, which only added to my fury. Why were they getting him involved in this when he so clearly didn't have the wherewithal to even understand the context of the argument in its entirety?!

"Oh, Colin, please don't worry about it. I don't blame you. I know you couldn't call me . . . I was just so worried about you. I am so sorry that I couldn't be there. I am so sorry; I love you . . . are you okay?"

"Yes, just tired. I'm going to go back to bed . . . is Pippa okay?"

"Yes, they say she's fine. We will be home hopefully by day's end. Is there anything I can do to help you?"

"No, just come home," was all he could muster before he said goodbye and I heard the phone disconnect.

Pippa and I returned home to find Colin sick and vomiting. She was still unwell too, and the house was as quiet as I can remember it ever being. Matthew, Tayt, and Jake had long since gone to bed; my mother had headed home; and I laid next to Colin, not sleeping—just watching him.

The next two days were filled with recovery and me moving from room to room, from Pippa to Colin. On the third, I awoke to found Colin out of bed. At first I panicked, wondering where he was, until I heard his voice downstairs. I heard him and Pippa in the kitchen: I heard him laughing, and then Pippa laughing and saying "Dada", and I realized that it wasn't a dream. (So many times over the past several weeks I had happened upon a similar scene, only to wake up and it was all a dream, wiping the sweat off of my brow and promising myself never to take anything for granted.) I lay in bed just a short while longer: eyes closed, relishing the moment, considering the possibility that I could someday have my life back. Colin came in to grab his baseball cap. He was still in his pajamas, but was looking strong.

"Hey, Jules, what do you want to do today?"

"Oh, I don't care. What do you want to do?"

"Well, really just one thing. I think I should go see my mom."

A feeling of nausea hit me when I heard him say that. I had been so immersed in playing nursemaid that I had completely blocked the entire scene out of my mind, if for only a brief period of time.

Minutes later, as I stood in the shower, letting the water wash away those painful events, Colin had a request for me.

"Jules, I need you to come with me to my mom's. I need for you two to make up. I need for it to be okay between the two of you. Please, if I am going to be able to focus on getting better, you are going to have to see her. Can we please get this over with today?"

"Of course, Colin." This was the VERY last thing that I wanted to do on this beautiful day—when, for the first time in a month and a half, life seemed worth living again—but he needed me to do it. He had asked me and, at that time, I would have gone to the ends of the earth to do what he needed. I would have given my own life to save his. And if this was one thing that he needed in order to save himself, then I would kiss her feet, wash her bathroom, whatever it took. I would eat crow, apologize, beg, if it would help keep him here with me, help bring him back to me.

I took my time getting out of the shower, and when I came downstairs everyone was at the table eating. Taytem's nurse Dorothea was there to take care of the kids as we went to make amends at Colin's parents' house. I knew that Colin had called them to tell them we were on our way, but I didn't know the extent of what was said: whether he had made the same plea to her; whether he knew the significant damage that had been done in his absence, the anger that I spewed. I have to say that, for the first time, I wasn't afraid. I was ready for the challenge. I was more than willing to go talk, perhaps meet in the middle, be prepared to move on—hopefully not having to apologize, but willing to do so if I had to.

We arrived at his parents' house. Ben met us at the door and asked us to have a seat in the two chairs at the front. In came Diana, all dressed in white, her hair standing up on end, still in her robe. She was visibly trying to hold back from racing across the room and ripping my head off. I looked at Colin, only to realize that he didn't have a clue of the carnage that was left in his wake. He looked completely oblivious to the amount of hurt and anger that was welling up all around him in that room.

We all sat silently, and then Diana started the conversation, sitting right in front of Colin and me. Colin was at ease in his chair, one leg crossed over the other: again, *zero* idea of what was coming his way. Diana had opened the conversation saying something to do with Pandora's Box, and the next thing I knew she was on a roll. I don't remember the entire assault that was launched, but I remember "selfish, self-centered, and ungrateful" were just some of the many things she called me.

I just sat there, expressionless: almost ready to defend myself; but knowing Colin needed peace, so I would let it go and apologize when she was finished. But then Colin responded.

"This is your idea of being fair? An ambush? All those things you said, all those attacks. We are done . . . come on, Julie, let's go. We're not going to sit and listen to this anymore. Let's go."

He got up, moving faster than I had seen him move in weeks, and started toward the door, only to turn around and grab my hand. He squeezed it tight and led me right out the door.

I was in disbelief—that was not what I had expected *at all*. It wasn't that I didn't know Colin loved me, but when it came to his mother, he always either took her side or tried to make light of the situation. I felt like I had won the battle. No matter what happened between Diana and me, I knew he would always have my back. The war was over: she could do and say anything that she wanted going forward, because she could never change our relationship. She was no longer a threat to my security. There was part of me that almost felt sorry for her in all of it. It was over for me: no more anger. Just the security that I had so desperately needed from the start, the security of knowing that Colin and I were truly one. If we could withstand his mother, if he was willing to stand by my side and to deny everyone around him, that was all that I needed.

When we arrived back at ours, Dorothea told us that Diana had tried to stop by before we had made it home, to apologize. I recognized in that moment that she could be upset with me: she was not MY mother. I also realized, being a mother myself, that this was not the time for her relationship with her son to fall apart. As angry as Colin was with her, I was not willing to be the rift that would form in his last days. I put myself in her shoes and told Colin that neither of us were thinking rationally, as illness does that to you. After discussing it for a bit, Colin's anger turned to acceptance, as it always did, and we never brought it up again. We all just put it behind us.

Chapter 17

This is my first blog, so please forgive me for my grammar. I want to thank all of you for your time, money, and kindness over the last 2 months. A month ago I was in such a drug coma to get over the pain and emotional time of learning of the cancer, that I really didn't realize the medical gravity I was dealt. A month ago, I couldn't get out of bed due to the abdominal pain without heavy painkillers. But in the last two weeks, my pain has decreased tremendously. I have energy to make it through the day with a couple naps. I can help Julie around the house and with the kids as much as most dads. I've been really optimistic about this turn in health. I just ended my first three weeks of chemo at the University of Chicago. After the first one I had unforgiving nausea. The last two were like having a light flu. I believe that the chemo has reduced my tumors and relaxed the abdominal area. This isn't a doctor's diagnosis, but I can feel it. When I take deep breaths, sneeze, or cough, I can feel that there is something wrong around the liver and pancreas. It feels like bad indigestion stuck in your lower chest. The day I can sneeze without feeling that pain will be day I know my health has returned.

JULIE BARTH

The first page of this website paints a pretty black future for our family. Not many people survive from pancreatic cancer. But I have received several messages from people that are beating the cancer or are in remission. It can be beaten and I'm very confident in my body to heal itself. I am working with acupuncture and holistic healing to give every chance for my body and brain to fight this battle.

Lastly, I haven't seen the total of the donations yet, but I know that they are more than I ever imagined. You have given me a great opportunity to fight the cancer without worrying about my financial stability over the holidays. Not many cancer patients are given this chance, and I will use this as motivation to fight every day. I will blog 1-2 times a week. The next big test will be a CT scan Jan. 17. Once I get any new info it will be posted.

Colin Barth

*

Tuesdays became "chemoday". We would wake up at six a.m. and head downtown to the University of Chicago for the all-day event. I'd thought we would go together and have some quality time—time to hang out, to talk, to reconnect. I thought it would be the perfect solution for that which we were losing by not being able to go out to dinner and spend the time alone as we used to. But, that very first time, I realized that the version of illness that we are fed on television: with those quality moments . . . well, in our world of sickness, it did not exist. Colin would be nauseous and vomiting the entire ride there. On the first trip, we exited the highway to go to the hospital (which was in a severely bad part of town, with a bail bondsman and pawn shop on every corner), and Colin looked at me with tears streaming from his eyes. He was ashamed to ask or put me out to stop, yet pleaded with his eyes for me to pull over. I did so just in time for him to exit the car and find a trash can on the side of the street, where he began to purge the McDonald's that, earlier on the way down, he had thought was a good idea. There were three men hanging out on the corner, who saw him and began to mock him: yelling things at him, probably assuming he was drunk. I didn't dare say anything, or even acknowledge them. I just wanted Colin to get back into the car, and quickly, so we could reach the safe zone of the hospital. Most of the time Colin would sleep while I drove; then, when we got there, he would play on his iPhone and then sleep again. I would use my BlackBerry to write our story, emailing it back to myself to then piece together once I got home.

We would sit in the waiting room, and when he was called up Colin would march in to take his poison. I swear I could see the blood drain from his face and body. After the "life-saving" poison would begin, he would turn an off-yellow shade. The ride home for him was the same as the ride down: the most uncomfortable-seeming sleep I could ever imagine. It would be marred by tremors, talking, mumbling under his breath, his lips and limbs moving. It was so hard to watch; there was not a peaceful moment to be found.

After two rounds of chemo in six weeks, he went in for another MRI to measure whether the tumors had shrunk or stayed the same. Following the first round, I'd started to see a slight improvement in him—in his spirit, in his strength, and in his pain levels. He stayed around more of the time, and at certain points the old Colin could be witnessed for a glimpse, before he would then go back to bed.

It was almost Christmas when he had his first scan. He went in at eight a.m.. He was actually well enough to go down by himself, and I think he needed to have a little independence back. He returned from it early and said that he would be receiving the results at the next chemo round. He headed back upstairs and went to sleep. Two hours later, when I went to check on him, I noticed that he was red all over and he was sitting up miserably, itching everywhere. It was the I realized the rash that he had in the hospital for the blood clots was caused by the MRI—he was allergic to the dye from the procedure. I called the doctor, who added another couple of medications to his list, which was becoming longer and longer over time.

It was nerve-racking and miserable, waiting for the test results. We had to sit through the entire chemoday and then just stay and wait to see Dr. Kinler. We were scheduled at the very end of the day, and it had already been a particularly long one. Colin looked like he would pass out from standing up. I said a silent prayer—probably for the first time since his diagnosis. So much rested on this moment and on these tests; so much of what we would hear that afternoon would change our lives. Of course, our lives had already been changed immeasurably, but this trial had given us the gift of hope—something that no one had given us since the day they found the tumor. From the moment the ER doctor came in to give him the news about the cancer, you could see it in everyone we encountered, you heard it at every turn: it was terminal.

This study and combination of drugs: this was it. This was the only option we had; this was the only hope that we could cling to. If we walked into that room to hear the doctor say that there had been no change, or—God forbid—that the tumor had grown or spread, then the hope that we needed so desperately to cling to, the hope that we were so much in need of, would be gone, and we would know that it was over, that this was the end of the ride.

At four p.m., we walked over to Dr. Kinler's office and were quickly escorted into a waiting room. Within moments, Dr. Kinler walked in. Although Colin had been signed up for the study, we had not seen her since that very first meeting.

"Hi, Colin, it is so good to see you. You look better; are you feeling any better?"

"A little," he whispered, barely able to find the energy.

"I was so thrilled to see that you were able to make it into the study, and you can thank Lauren for getting you in. She really went to bat for you when someone signed before you; she really fought to get you in."

Since Colin didn't know the story, I thought he would be puzzled. But, as I looked at him, I realized he didn't care about any of it; it was all going over his head. He just wanted to get the results and go home.

"So I hear you are allergic to the dye? We will have to pre-medicate for that next time."

"Okay."

Again, Colin could not have cared less.

"Well, Colin, I looked over your scans, and I am glad to say that your tumors have shrunk significantly . . . it is not at all what we expect on the first round. Normally there is not much or any shrinkage the first time at all, but your scans have shown that the tumor has been reduced twenty-four percent—that is truly amazing. It is very, very good, and it makes us very hopeful that you will do really well with this combination of drugs."

I was numb. I didn't know how to react. If I smiled, it would make light of the situation; if I didn't, I wasn't happy enough. So I sat frozen. Finally, I looked at Colin, who was expressionless, and knew I had to break the silence.

"What does that mean for next time?" I asked. "I mean, what would you expect to see happen next time?"

"Well," she began, "I think that for the next scan we would be looking for the tumors to maintain their size. I think to hope for more shrinkage might be a little unrealistic. I am surprised at what we saw today as it is. This is good news, Colin." She patted him on the back. "Really good news."

"Yeah, that's great," he said faintly, sounding either as if he wasn't as impressed, or he wouldn't allow himself to get excited. Or perhaps, after the long day, he really couldn't care less. He picked up his jacket, and I looked at him.

"Do you want me to go and get the car and pull it around?"

I was instantly aware that, unless they had said "That's it; all gone!", he knew in his heart that the battle we were waging had just begun; and, although we had gotten incredible news, it just meant more poison for him, more months of doing this, more cancer. The fact remained that he still had terminal cancer, and NO ONE was saying that there would ever be a time when he would live without it.

"No, I can walk with you," he said as he put his jacket on, "but I have to get something to eat."

We got into the car and exited the parking lot. After several minutes of total silence, he spoke.

"That's good news, isn't it, Jules? I mean, that's better news than we could have hoped for, right?" I let him just talk out loud, not daring to answer. I could see he was trying to feel comfortable with being excited; getting his hopes up for the first time in a long time. "I mean, I would have been happy with her saying that it hadn't spread . . . this is really good news, isn't it?"

After that, I became wrapped up in trying to save our home and trying to save money. The community had been fantastic, and had really come out to help and support us. The fundraising efforts in particular had been amazing. They had raised a lot of money; even opening up an account and putting enough in it to allow us to survive the next year if we had to.

Colin came to me shortly after Christmas and said to me that he really needed to get out of here. And so then we decided to take a family vacation to the beach. Being the control freak I have learned I am, I insisted on driving all of the almost twenty-six hours. We had decided to take my mother on the trip. Regardless of the fact that my mother hates nothing more than the beach, and is not too fond of warm weather, our prevailing thought was that she would be of tremendous help. My mother was trying so hard to wait and gauge what I needed from her, that it felt more like abandonment sometimes, so I asked her to come along. I don't think she would have let it play out any other way. Colin had had his chemo on Tuesday. We picked up the RV on Thursday, giving him a day and a half to recover, and on one of snowiest days of the year (for a moment fearing we were not going to even get out of Chicago!) we all jumped in and started our journey to Florida. The trip was hard: the kids spent the entire time throwing up and crying! They were all still so young. Even though Colin tried his hardest to rest and to heal from the chemo, it just didn't work that way. Every time I looked at him, he looked that same pale yellow, with no blood in his face. He was so very, very sick.

The trip down was one that I insisted on making fast, and I drove straight through. We ended up in Florida twenty-three hours later, parked the RV, and were by the cottage pool, sunning ourselves that very first day. Colin spent the first four days there in bed, while I myself spent the first three juggling the kids at the beach and at the pool. Colin came out for only an hour or two a day. On day five, he finally emerged from the bedroom with some energy, and was able to join in with the fun. With only two days left, we decided to stay an additional weekend and drive back to make it home in time for his next chemo.

Those last additional days were so much fun. Colin and I were somewhat on edge, but the kids didn't notice. It was exactly what we needed. It was necessary that we had my mother with us, but all of us being crammed into one space was a bit much! The kids were all missing Colin, and were busy just being kids; and Mom, who is not equipped with a whole lot of patience, was already tired, and already stressed out.

For my part, I hadn't even suggested that Colin and I spend some time together. I wasn't exactly afraid of him, but I was afraid of being alone with him—as it would force me to face the truth, the sadness, of realizing what I myself was missing. The only time that I really felt the loss of him—the only time I truly allowed myself to see what I was missing—was when I was with him. Then I was not really "with him", as partners, as we had been. When we did have time alone I was overcome with two emotions: one was the realization that "Colin and Julie" were gone forever. "Colin and Julie" were not just a couple; we were one person. You almost didn't utter one of our names without the other's. You know: like when you are a couple for so long, you lose your ability to be an individual. You become only a team. And so now, when we were out together, I realized that I needed to rediscover who "just Julie" was. Secondly, I didn't want to face the fact that he might not be around much longer. As long as I ignored it, I could do the daily routine: take care of the kids, pretend that I was working around him, and that I was waiting for the time he was going to be better. When we were together, I could see we were never going to be together in the sense that I could remember. My memories were fading away, and giving way to the "new us". I didn't want them to, I wanted to hold onto the "old us".

He had arranged before we left, not even knowing he would be capable come that point, for us to drive to the other island, just one over from Captiva. I hadn't even realized that he had given a single thought to anything other than trying to survive, but he had: he had wanted to have some time alone with me, with his wife; for, as much as I longed to avoid him, he longed to be with me. The island was famous for a lot of reasons, but mostly for the sunrise. Something about sunsets had always made him fascinated, made him feel alive.

Colin seemed more lighthearted than I had seen in months. He bought us T-shirts to remember our night out. He even bought me a drink, which I guiltily accepted while he drank O'Doul's. We made our way to the beach to watch the sunset and wait for our table. There were people everywhere, waiting just as we were for the sunset, sharing the same scene. Only I was fully aware that everyone around us had no idea of the significance of the sunset that we were watching. I became keenly aware that probably no one else around us felt the same sensation—that of their sunsets being numbered.

Colin grabbed his iPhone, brought it over to a random older couple near us, and asked if they would take our picture. Normally I would have shied away, asked that we not take one, but I saw in his eagerness that he needed this. The man agreed to take our picture. Colin put his arm around me, and for the first time in a very long time, we were connected. Then Colin handed me the camera.

"Here, now take a picture of just me and the sunset."

"Seriously?" I asked, kind of surprised that he would want just a picture of himself.

Later, looking at the pictures that I had taken, I became aware that Colin knew in his soul that his days were numbered. As much as we both kept up appearances, as much as he had pronounced that he was going to beat this, he had not truly believed it. He knew that his time was very limited, so he was leaving behind a present for us: the present of him and the setting sun. More importantly, he knew how vital it was to have that picture of him happy. I knew that was his intention; and that was the very last time that I can remember him smiling, laughing, full of life.

The trip home was less enjoyable than the trip there. There was a lot of throwing up, yelling, crying—the whole idea of taking an RV seemed ridiculous come this point. We'd had to park it the moment we got on the island, and, just like in the movie *National Lampoon's Vacation*, we returned to find that someone had taken all of our hubcaps! I knew the trip home was going to be as arduous as the one there, and Colin had not fared so well first time round. I tried to convince him to buy a ticket and fly home so we could just meet him there, but he was fearful of me going it alone, and although my mother was with us sometimes she added more stress than assistance. My mother is one of dearest women I have ever known, but not much of a go-getter. Colin had wanted for me to enjoy the vacation, but saw me running around more than being able to just sit and spend time.

After finally rolling into our driveway, I began to unload the RV. And at that moment my mother started just going off on Matthew. She had really been targeting him on this trip; and perhaps with good reason, as he was not behaving very well. But Colin and I knew what was behind his acting up—we could see the pain in his eyes. And so on this occasion that she started in on him, Colin had had enough. I was busy ferrying the suitcases into the house, and came outside to hear the profanities flying.

"Fuck you, Janet . . . he has said thank you more times in the past five minutes than you have said this entire trip . . . you sat on your ass."

I wanted to stop it, and I wanted to be on my mother's side. But looking at Colin, and seeing his need to be able to express his feelings to her, I was keenly aware that this situation was no different than the one that had occurred just a few short months ago between his mother and myself. I realized that perhaps we had to affirm to one another that we would each stand behind the other. I stood there on the porch as Colin was laying into her. She turned, only to see me there, inactive; glaring at me, as if to say "Do something. Are you just going to stand there and let him talk that way to me?" Although I wanted to step in; to keep the peace as one does; to say "Colin, that's enough", I didn't. Furthermore, the weather outside was awful. We had left Chicago in the middle of a snowstorm to return home to what had continued to be several days of more snowstorms, and some icing over to boot. Her car had sat in our driveway the entire week, so it was buried and stuck in ice. After Colin had let rip, he brought in the rest of the luggage and escaped upstairs. My mother walked through the front door as I was putting the food that was left away in the cooler.

"Your husband—" she started.

I looked up and said:

"Colin was right, Mom. You didn't say thank you once."

"Well, fine then. I will just go. I thought I was doing you the favor," she said, almost like she was waiting for me to come to my senses and to jump to her rescue. "And then he said that I was lazy and overweight, and that I don't take care of myself."

I looked at her again. "You know what, Mom, you don't. He has told you you need to take better care of yourself. He's dying, Mom, and he just wants you to take better care of yourself."

She grabbed her keys and headed to her car. I suppose I should have followed her, but I didn't. I didn't move to comfort her, to show my allegiance, to acquiesce to her insistence that he was wrong.

In an instant she was gone. I stood, not moving, continuing to put the food away in the refrigerator. Yet in just as short a time she was back again: like in a bad sitcom, when someone makes their grand exit and then has no choice but to come back because they forgot something.

"I need your phone," she muttered, anger underlying her utterance. "My car is stuck and I'm going to call a tow truck."

In that moment, although I refused to comfort her, I also pitied her and loved her and felt sorry for her.

"No, Mom, that's ridiculous. I'll help you."

"I am just going to call a tow truck," she shot back.

I went out to find her in her car, apparently intending to sit there all day, so I got down and just started to push. I pushed and she hit the gas. We worked simultaneously, both of us wanting her to be able to go home and cool down, without intervention. This went on for about ten minutes, and just when I believed that we would have to call for assistance, she backed up one more time, hit a patch of something where she found traction, and off she went. The only thing I saw was the back of her car and the ridiculous hat she wore as she made her way home. I returned inside, put the remainder of the vacation packing away and the situation with my mom to one side, and went to check on Colin, who was sound asleep. After watching him, peaceful, I myself experienced one of those rare moments of quiet rest. Then Pippa started to cry, and the world returned. We were home, things were back to normal. Well, as normal as they had been when we left.

Colin asked me several times after that vacation for us to go away together, as a couple. I always made an excuse to not. I still feel the sting of guilt when I picture him asking. I couldn't handle being alone with him: it would be too much, it would have broken my soul. I wasn't capable of being that close, that raw, that honest, to spend time alone with him—with no distraction, no children, to pull me back into life. I was fearful of living in his world, in his fear, in his suffering.

*

I often pray to Colin wherever he is that he will be able to forgive me for not having the strength to spend the time with him that he so desperately needed; the time that he longed for. Living without such forgiveness is something that will rob your soul of the ability to move on, to live again. For just one brief moment I wish that he could hear me, to understand the sincerity in my apology, and my shame, and most importantly my devastation that I didn't ever go, that I didn't spend the time with him when *he* had the strength, when *he* was good.

I missed out on the time that I thought I would have forever. You always think "tomorrow", but tomorrows sometimes don't come. There are so many times and so many things that I mull over lately, as if wishing I could say aloud or straight to Colin that I want to apologize for so many things I could change.

*

After returning from the trip, he had begun communicating with the children again, and with me again. And so after chemo we would go for lunches. They were quiet and calm, but we would again have (albeit slight) pieces of conversation about the life we shared together, the kids, the house, and he began to demonstrate some positivity, some feeling that he might be around to care about the future.

As Colin and I were sitting at a restaurant during one such meal, we were both focusing heavily on the plates in front of us. We weren't avoiding each other; I suppose we were more just appreciating the silence and time alone. Then a whisper escaped his mouth.

"Julie, what do you think it is that kills you when you have cancer?" He looked up from his plate now, and then across to me. "I mean, I know you die of cancer . . . but what do you think it is about the cancer that you actually die from?"

I was trying with all my being to not look shocked or devastated, to not show how I felt inside—my heart breaking at the mere mention of him dying.

"Well," I started, very cautiously, "I would think that the cancer affects your body in a way that destroys its functioning . . . I suppose when the cancer finally destroys the organs to the point where they no longer function, I think that is probably what kills you."

I said this in the most matter-of-fact way. I knew that he needed to let me know that he was thinking about death—that he was pondering the fact that he might not beat this. He knew what he was up against, and although everyone in our world would shrug off the seriousness of the situation (during any mention of the cancer, the serious subject of death would be swerved via either pretending that it wasn't happening, or that he was going to beat it), no one was allowing him to entertain the notion that he might die. I thought in that moment that all of us were doing him an injustice: to not recognize the potentiality of his death, to shrug off the severity of the situation. I knew that not only did he need to face it, but he needed me to deal with it, to see that it might not go the way we wanted. He needed to know that I could handle it, and that I understood that he might not make it.

He looked deep into my eyes, as if searching for how I felt—he needed affirmation of one kind or another—and then he set his gaze back onto his plate, and the silence lingered until the conversation turned to something meaningless: like getting the Jeep fixed, or the mundane chores required to get the house back into order.

He accepted my analysis of what could happen, and he never asked again. He never questioned whether I was right. That intense recognition of him, looking so deeply into his eyes, was something I hadn't realized I had ceased to do. Looking at him had become painful because I forever continued to look for the self-assured and calming eyes that I loved and needed. When I searched and could no longer find them, I stopped looking at all.

Colin continued with the chemo—Tuesdays; three weeks on, one week off—into the spring. He was in a tremendous amount of pain, and would spend most of his time locked away in our bedroom. On good days, or days when he had the week off, he would find time to come down and help me, if only for a short while. He found great satisfaction in really doing nothing else but feeling useful and available to me.

Jake had been on a traveling team the year before Colin's diagnosis, and the other team members and their parents had become somewhat of a family to us all. This is what happens when you spend as much time as we did together—watching your children grow together; working together to get them somewhere; carpooling, even your weekends and your nights usually spent together. Jake was starting up baseball again in the spring, and, with Colin beginning to feel slightly better, it seemed like someone had breathed a little life back into our world. Pippa was now a year old, and just full of the devil (as she is now, and as she always will be!); Taytem was quiet and shy and just finishing up her kindergarten year. That year that was filled with the blessings of uneventfulness. Not once in that entire time during the winter and into the spring did Taytem get sick or require hospitalization. Rather, she seemed to flourish.

Now that I knew that there really wasn't anything I could do for her, good or bad, that knowledge in itself removed such a heavy burden. And although I was dealing with Colin's illness, when it came to Taytem I had found a new freedom, and in her I saw a little light shining. I no longer felt the need to put her in a bubble, and seclude her from the world. She needed to be untied from my apron strings and she was soaring. Where once my story was all about Taytem—traveling, doctors, therapies, constantly trying to "fix" whatever I saw wrong with her—I found peace with her situation. You know that phrase "God only gives you what you can handle"? First, let me clear up my stance on that, in that I would disagree. I have been given way more than I can handle—many, many times. But in this instance, it was almost as if whomever is in charge of the universe decided to give Tayt a break. As Colin's illness progressed, hers seemed to ameliorate, or perhaps it was as if I wasn't focusing so much on her; her past, her future. I was just letting Tayt for the first time in her life "do Tayt". She did have occasional health issues throughout the months that Colin was sick, but they seemed less immediate, less overpowering, less all-consuming. Maybe it was that she was getting better and stronger, or maybe it was that I couldn't throw the energy I once did at her, it was now being dispersed. Ironically, it was in my inability to focus all of my attention to and on her that she found the independence she not only needed, but she probably had been longing for, for a long time.

And so that spring we spent hours and hours on the ball field. It's just you and the rest of the parents: watching, engrossed, catching up with the others around you, bonding over shared misfortunes or your dislike of the other team. Colin enjoyed hanging out with the other dads, but it wasn't like the old days. Traditionally he would stand there, quite obviously one of the tallest dads, and most likely the most boisterous; unable to keep out of things, incapable of keeping his opinions to himself, engaging everyone around him. This season was different. Colin, whose pants were now hanging halfway down his butt (he always refused to purchase new pants, thinking he would grow back into them), would just pace. He would chew gum and he would pace. He started to hang back from the other guys, not really engaging, and his comments were few and far between. His jovial attitude had become more serious, and his demeanor of helpfulness now seemed to be more one of frustration. He tried to help more with the kids during games, perhaps to convince himself that things were still the same. While I sat in the stands watching, he would take Matthew and Pippa off to a nearby park to busy himself. He missed the banter and didn't even have the energy to engage; it was easier to avoid the game altogether. His absence was felt and changed the entire team. If he came, he would leave me sitting alone in the stands. The changes in him were superficial to everyone else and the smile that we both wore when we were out betrayed what was happening inside our home: how the illness had been swallowing us whole. The entirety of "us" was being sucked away, leaving "us" a shell of what everyone else wanted to see. And that was exactly it: everyone wanted to know how

I was feeling, how it was going; but, when I would reply, unless it was positive, or fine, I would instantly get a look from them, like that of a deer caught in the headlights. So I resorted to saying that everything was fine. I felt continually like a traitor to our cause if I let the guard of him being simply perfect down. It was a betrayal to him to admit that he might not make it.

The guys on the baseball team didn't see it, or else couldn't handle it, or simply didn't know what to do. But I think Colin felt more like they had left him behind, like they had forgotten him. He would avoid them, and although they didn't know why, it was due to the sheer feeling of loss he had when he was with them. Much like I didn't feel the full effect of missing his presence after he got sick, he was able to pretend the world had melted away and didn't exist. Everyone is around you, watching you sink. If you fuss, if you move, it only makes the despair feel greater—so you hold still, you hope it will all go away. To watch you suffer is too much, so the majority walk away; but those left—the ones you feel should pull you out—eventually become frustrated. They can no longer stand the suffering, and they too walk away, but it is the moments prior to them just walking away that hurt the most. It is seeing them continue as normal: living life, living in the same world, continuing to enjoy and to smile and to live, to make new connections, new friends, form new memories, new ties, right in front of you—as you watch on: stuck, sick. You know realistically there is nothing they can do. (If they jump in with you, you will both surely go down; it will take you both.) But the jealousy of wishing to be on the outside, and the guilt of them watching from the inside, destroys all involved. Your head tells you that they had to move on; they had to continue to live; they had to find a way to live without you around; they can only stay too long before they realize that them just trying to remain close, to keep an eye on you from a short distance, is even more tortuous. And they realize in the end that, for so many complex reasons, they too must walk away, leave you to sink, leave you to suffer alone, in order to save themselves.

Colin and I had been two halves of a whole our entire adult lives, and been in one another's lives as long as I could remember. And then it was like one day, he was just gone. As couples, there are those deep, secret, and intimate conversations you have about your feelings and your pain. But those stopped for us. The last thing that I could do is go to Colin and complain about the isolation I was feeling; the anger I was trying to swallow at everyone seemingly ignoring that I needed help. I did not want to make his burden more. At the very worst moments of my life, when I needed my best friend more than I could have ever imagined, he was not available. I couldn't talk to other people about how I felt—that almost seemed like a betrayal of Colin and his trust. He was doing everything he could to keep up the appearance that he was "fine". He needed to live in the fantasy that he was fighting and winning and going to make it. If I told people what was truly going on behind closed doors—the suffering, the vomiting, the crying out in pain that never stopped—it felt like I was selling him out, ruining the facade that he needed to keep. At the same time, however, I needed for people I knew to know what he was dealing with, what I was dealing with. It all seemed an act. My life was no longer mine. I was living in the "Colin's Illness" story and I was only a supporting character. But you say things like that, and before your brain can process the words yourself, you want to get them out of your head—as if someone will see them and judge you for them, think you a bad person.

All the while, Colin, who I am sure needed his best friend too, was not going to burden me with his fears, his pain, his need to talk about death, possibilities, after he was gone; his guilt for leaving us on our own. He didn't say much about anything. He avoided any visitors. he was silent. It was like he was hiding within, where no one could touch his desire to avoid and ignore the inevitability of what might happen. It's funny: at a time when you would think you would want to lean on your spouse or loved one the most, it is when you begin to pull back—like two negatives might take you both down.

Colin would get super dressed-up for the smallest events. A couple of times, he went to the tanning booth, not wanting to look too pale. If we had somewhere to go, he would spend the day before preparing his outfit and mustering up the energy to be outgoing. The day after, he would disappear to recuperate from all the effort it took. I would hear over and over "Colin looks great" and just nod, not wanting to spill the secret that it wasn't real and that he was faking it. The worst part? I was angry at him too. All the energy he put into making people think he was okay was robbing me, the kids, the people who really missed him, of time with him. I was upset that he was giving to others what I felt should be mine. All of the months he spent fighting cancer and, maybe as importantly, fighting the appearance that he had cancer or that it might be winning, he never talked to me about how he was feeling inside. Like I didn't want to hear what my brain was thinking, he didn't want to talk aloud about what was happening, because then it really would be. But then I felt guilt again for being upset that he chose to put his energy into things I thought were unimportant. Illness fucks everything up, period.

Colin had gone through another cycle of chemo and then had a scan. And we were so over the moon when they told us that his tumors had shrunk *another twenty-three percent*. There were not many days after that initial diagnosis that Colin was so jovial and the mood was so light. We were joking around, laughing, teasing each another—it was one of the very few times that I actually enjoyed accompanying him. The couple of weeks leading up to it had been like a breath of fresh air, too, as the chemo had been mild and his response had been minimal. We had almost begun talking about a time when he didn't have cancer. We felt like we were almost there: so close that we could almost reach out and touch it. So when Helen had come in with her assistant and given us the miraculous, wonderful news, it only added to the existing sense of elation that we had brought with us that day.

On the way home we actually dared to dream. We talked about a time when he could go for surgery. And then this narrative just kept getting fuller the longer we drove. We talked of a time for him to return to work, a time of more children, of a life away from and outside of this cancer world. We were for the first time really and truly imagining and believing in a time when we could return to our lives: a time when Colin would be healthy and happy and *living* again.

With Colin getting the good news also came a decision. At the time it seemed like a minor one, but Jake—who was turning eleven—was supposed to go to a tournament in Omaha. Only guys were going:

the boys and their dads. Unfortunately, it came during an "on" week, and so, if Colin chose to travel, he would be taking more than a week off chemo. He insisted that it was that important for him to go, and although I was very fearful I understood his thought process. He and I both knew how incredibly important this trip was: not only to Jake, but to Colin. Now, with this good news that we had received, there was absolutely no talking Colin out of it. Yet I don't know why I felt as panicked as I did. I couldn't talk him out of it, but something inside me sensed he shouldn't go. With Colin's being so excited, and so adamant, I felt the need to stand behind his decision; and, as I kissed him goodbye, I prayed silently that I was mistaken and that this truly was the right thing to do. Though, in the pit of my stomach, something was very, very wrong.

From the moment he got back from that trip with Jake, I knew something had changed. And as the weeks progressed, he started experiencing more pain. About a month on from his return, I begged him to just go to the doctor and alert someone of his suffering. One day in late summer, Colin decided that he was going to go into the hospital for chemo and not return home until they had figured a way to get his pain under control. If they could keep him in the hospital and put him on IV drugs to curb the pain, then they could come up with a better plan of treatment and create a home regimen to minimize his pain.

He took off for chemo all by himself, feeling well enough to take this on his own. He called me as soon as he had been admitted. I felt so completely helpless and guilty. I knew that I should have been with him. He must have felt so alone, but he never complained or made me feel like my priorities were in the wrong place. I called him several times over the day "just to check in". He sounded in good spirits and said that they were doing what they could to control the pain. He named medications like Dilaudid, morphine, methadone, Lyrica—they were throwing it all at him. Though he sounded at times completely coherent, at others it was like he was on a different planet. During his last call, he said that he missed me and really wished that I could come and stay with him. That was my cue to suck it up and go to him. So I did. I found a sitter and hopped into the car to drive downtown.

Chapter 18

Tuesday was another day of excruciating pain, trying to shake the stupor that was induced, for a while I was somewhat afraid he had suffered some sort of stroke. Wednesday was enough, we went to seek a second opinion at a hospital closer to home where we met with a man who I tell you no lie, when I tell you showed us more compassion and humanity than this journey has afforded up until now. To make a long story short, he clued us into the fact that Colin has cancer growing on his T11 vertebrae ... we don't know whether it has been there from the get-go, just completely shocked that we saw, oh I don't know, 20 different doctors, who omitted that information in the hospital stay that did nothing but rob more time from me and our children ... so we decided to radiate the spot, and hopefully make the pain lessen, met with yet another pain doctor, who again, was a pleasure, sincerely, who gave Colin a shot in the neck and for the first time, he experienced some relief, even if for a brief period, he played football, ran around the field, spent time with Jake for the first time in months ... on Thursday he went downtown to resume chemo only to find out that not only had they omitted the information of the back, but because of that very information, he has been kicked out of the experimental study, and "don't bother coming back because we have nothing for you" . . . it is amazing the difference between research doctors and the doctors who are practicing, I suppose their motives in research are more global, but the feel is one of cold, cut throat, we love you when you are proving us right, you are gone when you are not . . . so, Colin will start radiation tomorrow, hopefully gain some alleviation from pain, and we are going to regroup and find another course.

I can't say it didn't come as a shock, a scare, and well a devastation that this treatment that has been seemingly saving his life is being withheld . . . I would be lying to say that this is not a setback, a frustration, it is, no doubt, it is . . . but we have been here before with Tayt, we are not new to setbacks, bad odds, harsh, cold doctors, bad medicine, yes, we have seen it all, we have fought through it all, and Tayt is here, she is happy, she is healthy . . . she is everything they said she WOULDN'T be and everything I always believed she would. Colin's dreams these days are filled with a few brief moments of uninterrupted sleep . . . he dreams of beaches, quiet vacations, us together, him not sick . . . I dream of Colin walking Pippa down the aisle (God willing anyone will ever put up with her long enough to marry her), watching Jake graduate . . . my dreams are of future, Colin's are of moments of bliss, I suppose they are both the same, I think it is just a testament of the pain he feels continually . . . for the first time today Colin said that his head didn't hurt, but he has spent all day throwing up and I said to him in jest "what do your body parts take turns torturing you . . . it's as if your head said, I'm tired, stomach can you take over", yes, my humor, to him . . . not so much.

He will start 10 days of radiation tomorrow, again, we are flying blind, no idea what to expect, what it will bring, but we are going to weather this storm ... for those of you who have had the opportunity to speak with Colin ... he continually will tell you that I saved his life ... I feel guilty when he says that because I am unable to truly save his life right now, but I will be damned if I am going to give up, stop trying or let him either. We were meant to fight this together, I just wish I could do more, find someone, anyone to say "I can make this go away", any cost would not be too much, any ... As I am writing this Colin is pacing the room, back and forth he paces trying desperately to find something, anything to make the pain go away for just a moment in time ... that is what MY dreams are for him a moment, a lifetime ... winning the war on cancer huh? I would hate to see what losing would look like ... I will keep you posted as the week progresses ... I just feel like I had to exonerate the pain doctors, they didn't nick his back, but the other doctors, well, they nicked our soul ... until another time ...

*

I walked down the corridor of this strange hospital floor. It was nothing like I was used to. After all those years of staying with Taytem, I was used to fingerprints on the walls, color-coded tape leading to the NICU or the PICU, bright colors, fish tanks, books, and toys all over. This hospital floor was so different from what I had pictured. Of course they didn't want bright colors or handprints. I instantly became aware that this hospital ward was to keep people comfortable. It had one goal and one goal only: to relieve people's suffering. As I got closer to Colin's room, I saw that he was out of bed and walking around. He had his IV pole with him, and was laughing and walking with one of his friends from the Board of Trade. He saw me and his face instantly lit up. There were very few occasions lately that I saw his heart light. In that moment, I had a flashback of who he used to be. It was both a blessing and a curse. He immediately made a U-turn and headed to me in the hallway.

This ward was the last-ditch effort to be humane, to try to end the suffering that so many experienced as the catalyst to moving on. The patients on this ward were being given medicine to die; they were on the last leg of the journey. Yet here was Colin: full of more life and more happiness than I had seen him exhibit in a while, just from seeing me. I had a wave of panic come over me at the mere prospect that we would one day be here for the true purpose for which it was created. I was so overcome, experiencing such mixed emotions: the joy of seeing Colin smiling, and the fear of where this disease might potentially take us.

"You're a sight for sore eyes," he said as he picked up speed, wheeling his IV pole down the hall in a hurry to see me. He gave me a huge hug and a smile.

"How are they treating you here?" I asked. "Are you feeling any better?"

"I think they're finally getting the pain under control," he answered. "They've given me methadone, and it really just freezes everything. I feel much better. I can still feel the pain and the tumor, but it doesn't hurt nearly as much . . . I think I might be able to come home today.

I was instantly aware of my misgivings at not having had the courage, nor the constitution, to have stayed here with him and to have been at his side for the past twenty-four hours. But in that present moment, in which he was also entertaining returning to work, and the banter and gossip of office politics was bringing him back to life, he was more animated than I had seen him in a while. The nurse popped her head round the door to check in and see what Colin needed. Colin began discussing where he was on a pain scale. He had, over the past twenty-three hours, bonded with this nurse: getting to know her, joking with her; and, been his sarcastic self, he began to introduce me to her, and her to me, as if they were old working buddies from years past. She had a huge smile on her face, and every question she asked him came back with a new level of sarcasm, all in good fun. By the time she left, it was almost like Colin had given her the armor with which to continue on down to the hall to deal with the not so good cases that she was certain to endure.

Colin was in such a hurry to get out of there and test out his new drug-induced comfort, that, as soon as he saw me, he packed his things and was ready to be given his walking papers. There was something about Colin—there always was, even up until the very end—whereby, whenever he saw my face, his smile lit up and his eyes shone. The way that he did this whenever I entered the room, whenever I showed up anywhere, sent butterflies to my stomach the way that no one else ever could, I was so glad that he was coming home.

However, the months of Colin's illness were starting to take their toll on me.

*

Anyone who has had tragedy in their lives knows that, when people ask how you are, what they really want to hear is some variation of "fine", else the conversation turns too serious. If it does, you soon see it in their face: it is as if someone sucked all the life out of the room. They start looking around nervously; they start finding excuses to force you to see the positive side of whatever you are telling them. Whatever horrible things you are dealing with, they need to make themselves feel better and more comfortable by saying things that they think will make you look on the bright side. They throw out phrases like "it could always be worse" or "he looks really good" or "I saw him the other day and he looks fantastic". I knew that they were neither testing me, denying me, nor believing that I was being untruthful—they were finding a way to help *themselves* deal with it.

Some people surprise you in the best possible way. A woman I to this day barely know still stops by, brings banana bread, and drops notes. In the dead of that same winter, I would show up to find that she had shoveled my porch. She saw a need and took the initiative.

Chapter 19

To anyone who knows me, really knows me, they know that I have an inability to keep my mouth quiet. As one of my friends commented, "you tell it like it is", I don't know if that's true, but I certainly tell you how I see it. I read Colin's obligatory blog, he wrote it to make everyone feel better, to make everyone stop worrying, feel better about his illness. In all fairness the reason I am compelled to write this is because I need to tell you what I see. I need to tell you the truth of the situation, not as we would like it to be, but the true story. I believe that is what a blog is for... we have been incredibly blessed. I often tell the story about how they told me from the get-go to take Colin home, call hospice and "enjoy the couple of weeks we had left", yes we have been incredibly blessed! But this blessing has not come at no cost to Colin... I could never have imagined at the beginning of this ordeal what he would endure in the last couple of months. I wouldn't thought it possible. Not that I thought it was going to be a fairytale existence, but I never once imagined the torture, the sheer agony of what I would experience his mind, body and soul to go through. When he said 40% of the time he is with us, that really meant 40% of the time that he is functioning, equals a very limited time. I have never seen anyone endure the amount of pain, the amount of agony, torture, relentless that this illness has brought him, never in a million years can I describe it. It would be, I suppose like describing 9/11 . . . how do you even try? It all seems horrible to us far removed, but to those that were there, well, it is unimaginable. That is the way Colin has "survived" the past couple of months . . . I sometimes feel like we are in a casino . . . we were at the winning table, all those scans coming back each with a new promise of cure, we kept rolling the dice and coming up aces. But, who hasn't sat next to those people whose aces stop coming, albeit, hopefully just for a while. Yes, we will switch tables and start again and hopefully have success, but the last scan, seeing no improvement, and watching the ordeal he has been through, it didn't equal out . . . it didn't make it appear worthwhile. His last scan showed minimal growth, but with it came a migraine, debilitating, blinding, dizzying headaches, only to be scared that it had spread to his brain.

So the Monday following chemo he went in for a scan of his brain to make sure that it hadn't spread. I was on pins and needles, Colin, didn't even care . . . to him, he didn't care what the reason, he just wanted it to stop. The scan came back normal, good news . . . bad news, no cancer, but the chemo is attacking all of his nerves . . . he can't feel his fingers, can't feel his toes, can't feel his teeth, I know he's alive right? . . . ugh . . . I don't mean to sound pessimistic . . . my time with Colin is not over, my time with Colin is precious . . . when he smiles it makes my soul soar . . . it makes me feel like anything is possible. My life has been built around my best friend . . . the perfect human being, to me . . . I can't remember a time when he wasn't with me, throughout all phases of my life he has been there, he is my existence.

So when he says he's fine, he's not, he's trying to make sure that you are fine with where he is at. When he says he's okay, he's not . . . when I read when he blogged, I anticipated giving my narrative, but I realized that you all want to know the truth. The truth is not comfortable, it is not fun, but it is what Colin deserves for everyone to know. He is carrying this burden, this burden of suffering, but minimizing it because that is who he is. I just want for one night for him to remember what it is like to go out, have a drink or two, talk with friends, enjoy the evening, not feel pain, if only for 4 hours, but that relief never comes . . . but there is no room for escape, nowhere for him to go . . . if you get a chance, please just drop him a note. Not only has this illness become tiresome, but it is beginning to feel very isolating . . . all of a sudden you notice that the phone has stopped ringing, the emails have stopped coming . . . yes, life has gone on for everyone, but Colin and I are stuck here in what Colin phrased as "Groundhog day". For him, nothing changes, just varying degrees of angst and pain . . . it's all too much, too much for any one person to deal with . . .

*

After that trip to Omaha, Colin began complaining about leg pain. *Terrible* leg pain. He was no longer able to sleep at night. One of the hardest things for Colin to deal with was that he was only able to sleep in one position, almost sitting up. I didn't realize at the time how debilitating it was to no longer be able to move any which way, to toss and turn. I once heard a statistic—probably untrue—that each of us change positions over one hundred times a night in order to get comfortable. But Colin was unable to move at all. No relaxation in his sleep, equalling no peace nor rest. I would wake in the middle of the night—sometimes seven times, sometimes perhaps as many as twenty—to find him pacing. He wore out our carpet doing it, literally. The nights got to the point where neither of us would sleep at all, and so the days became a time for him to catch up. But there was no catching up for me. I had four children, missing their father; I was working full-time, selling things on Ebay to pay our Bens; plus a life that I couldn't just say "Sorry, I'm tired" to: so I would drag my butt out of bed early every morning. I was burning the candle at both ends.

There is only so long you can keep up that pace, and that you can bury your true worries, your true feelings, insecurities, losses. I would begin to try to find a way to escape watching Colin suffer; to escape the realization that, without the old life that we had together, I wasn't enjoying the new one. I felt uncomfortable and fearful around him. I walked on eggshells: making sure not to say the wrong thing, not to look at him the wrong way. In hindsight it must have seemed like I was looking right through him, as if he was no longer there. To me, my Colin was no longer there, and the person who stood in front of me not only was different but was forcing me to see myself for who I really was.

Colin's dream of returning to work slowly started dwindling away. It was a goal that was disappearing in front of our very eyes. His time in bed increased, and although he was not one to complain, he frequently spoke about how much his legs ached. I was watching him slide further into pain and anguish. All the progress that we had fought so hard for in those first months seemed to have been ripped from us. The fragile, sick, tortured soul, who had left the hospital to come home and die all those months ago, was reemerging right in front of me.

Our home had become a medicine chest filled of incredibly high-caliber drugs—the kind that could kill Pippa if she so much as licked one. On a daily basis, and to my constant terror, I would find Pippa sailing down the hall with his prescription bottles in hand, shaking them like maracas. One time she got hold of his anti-nausea medication and there was red surrounding her mouth. I asked Colin how many had been in the jar, because when I found her with it there was only one left, and that had clearly been in her mouth. After a call to the poison control center, I had to rush her to the hospital for observation. I spent five hours in the emergency room, just to make sure that she was okay. It was an ongoing panic—endless nights full of nightmares that she had overdosed on his medications. As many times as I asked him to please not leave his medications lying everywhere, it was like talking to a child. He would forget; grabbing for a bottle when he was in extreme pain, and then leaving it sitting on the nightstand.

The bedroom had finally and officially become his cell. He was no longer my husband or anyone's "daddy". He was the prisoner of illness, kept locked up and away in our room. He stopped coming downstairs, he stopped talking to the kids, he stopped talking to me. The pacing, the foot shaking, and the misery only intensified. One day I found him sitting at the edge of the bed. He couldn't breathe; he was at the edge of the bed, gripping his heart, gripping his side in fear, and I finally said enough was enough. He had previously decided he no longer wanted to go to the hospital; whatever it was, he felt he could control it at home. But looking at him sitting there, gasping for air, I finally thrust the white flag into his hand and we went to the emergency room. After spending another night and day at the hospital, he was told that he had again developed blood clots. This time, however, they were running the length of his legs: from the top of his ankle to the top of his hip joint. If one of them had become dislodged, it would have killed him instantly.

During this time, there was a professor that Oprah was touting. Like Colin, he had pancreatic cancer and he knew it was terminal. He started writing seminars to tell people that death was not all that terrible. People began asking me if I had watched his last seminar—as if I was not already living it. (I was angered, thinking *I should be writing seminars*.) This professor, so excited was he by being given the gift of knowing the importance of his final days, was onstage, giving talks, traveling around the country. That was *not* Colin's experience. Colin was fighting it just as hard, but his experience was not one of seeing the greatness of life and the fragility and preciousness of it. His experience was of being in such unbearable pain that he could no longer talk to his children, leave his room, or have his life.

Everyone who had seen Colin in this period had commented on how good he looked. I suppose it was easier for everyone to believe that he was doing as well as he looked, and that I was exaggerating how sick he was. When people would say, "I saw Colin the other day—he looks great" I would respond by saying he looked better than he felt. I would launch into tirades about how badly he was doing: I would describe the pain, the hardship, the misery of the situation. Not because I wanted the pity, although I suppose I did need it at the time. I felt the need to tell people the story of what Colin was enduring. He was not standing on a stage, telling everyone that he was unafraid to die. He was not traveling around the world, doing pushups in front of an audience. He couldn't even go out without it exhausting him for days after.

The blood clots in Colin's legs were so severe that they had to surgically insert "drainage tubes" into his femoral veins. There was some issue with his anatomy, and, as was true of most of the things Colin endured, the procedure ended up being much more complicated (him having to have two tubes inserted instead of one). I sat in the waiting room as they transferred him for the procedure. Since he had been placed on so many heavy-duty blood thinners, the procedure was now a dangerous one. As they wheeled him past, I remember his eyes looking at me with such adoration, and me kissing him and saying that it would be alright. I think for the first time since his diagnosis, for the first time since this ordeal began, my prayers for him didn't revolve around or start with "please save him—please don't let him die". For the first time, I prayed for mercy for him. In my heart I felt that it didn't matter what the end result was. It was no longer about keeping him alive, praying for the cure, praying to keep him in my life. As they wheeled him away the guilt began growing in me. This is because I had begun to wish that perhaps something would go wrong; that he would find some relief: not through the procedure, but by not having to endure this pain, this tortuous journey, any longer. I began to pray for an end to this for all of us, most of all him. I knew that at this point to pray for more of this—more of him slipping away, more of my soul slipping away—I just couldn't do it anymore. The guilt was great, and perhaps still is. But, at that very moment, I prayed for an end to it, to all of it.

By this point my inner world became a constant state of guilt. I felt guilty that I dreamt of a day that the nightmare would be over; about moving on and finding a life outside of the hell that I was living. I felt guilty because I had lost pretty much all of my friends—my best friend to an illness I could do nothing to change, and the rest to an illness that was growing within me that I could no longer control. I felt guilty that I couldn't stand to see Colin in so much pain. I would go up two or three times a day, and would always see him in the same position (whether he was sleeping or awake, he was always in agony). He had a chair by the bedside. When he was having a particularly good day—which was almost never at this point—he would sit in it. He would just sit, shake, massage.

Colin's headaches had also increased tenfold since his return from the Omaha trip. It had taken more out of him than I think he or I realized. Most of the time the headaches would leave him bedridden, and with the lights out. As, although they were finally able to get the blood clots under control, and the drainage valves seemed to do their job—which was to keep the clots from traveling to his heart—the headaches proved to be more problematic than anything else we had encountered up until then. He would spend his days yelling at anyone who dared make their way into our room. Pippa, who was just a baby at this point and learning to walk, would make a beeline to our room any chance that she could to see him. Colin was the light of her life; he was the one who made her smile. But with the new blood clots and the headaches, he had retreated more and more into his own world, leaving her out of it. If she entered the room, he would just start yelling. At this point, he was taking so much medication that I am quite sure that not only did he not know he was yelling at her, but he really might not have even known it was her. Jake was the only one who was allowed into the room. Not only was he allowed; he was being summoned. Colin, who was feeling very isolated, had found comfort only in Jake's company. He wanted Jake to watch sports with him all the time. He had no use for me, either. If I entered the room, he would immediately come at me: angry about what I hadn't done, what hadn't worked to ease his pain, what I didn't bring, the breakfast that he couldn't eat . . . it went on and on. Otherwise, I would enter the room to be confronted with his guilt at missing the toilet while vomiting. In Colin's mind, his anger was due to not being able to help me out. He was so angry that he couldn't be the husband that he so desperately wanted to be—the husband he had always been. And it was so hard to see him struggle during this time. However, his anger was so deep—and the things that he would say to me, the way he would treat me: as if I didn't even exist anymore—it was so hard to overlook, to look past. I guess, just as my friends were having a hard time overlooking the anger that was being hurled at them, so too I was.

It is hard to be the caregiver to someone you love and watch them suffer. As I explained before, outside of our house we were making a good show of how well we were surviving. I was dancing so hard to distract attention from the fact that my world was falling apart. I was working overtime to hide the gravity of what we were dealing with from my kids, our family and friends, and perhaps—if I want to be honest—from me. I was not willing to accept that things weren't just magically going to be okay. It was as if I didn't acknowledge that my world was being ripped from me; that it must not be real. In an attempt to put on that show, however, I lost me. So busy trying to make everything comfortable for everyone else, I felt like a fake. I was lying to everyone, while at the same time pissed at everyone for not seeing what was I thought right in front of them. You can't fight hard to make sure you hide the truth and then get angry that people don't see truth. I began to carry my internal struggle with the real world on my sleeve. I was easily offended, even more quickly angered; and, to the outside world, it probably not only looked disproportionate to the situation. For someone who wasn't hearing all my self-talk; it most assuredly seemed to come out of nowhere. Being my friend was no longer easy, or, I would dare say, possible. I was falling apart, and doing everything I could to put a facade of "I'm so put together" to the outside world. At some point, something had to give. What gave were my friendships, the way that I saw myself and who I was, leading to an inability to be social that pushed people even further away.

The terrible headaches, which were thought to be another symptom of the blood clots, were becoming so severe that I could no longer stand and watch it continue. Colin was no longer eating; no longer acknowledging me; the kids were no longer allowed in our room; his communication with everyone had stopped. I begged him to go back to the hospital and to tell them that, again, he would not leave until they had solved the problem. Before this, he had received what they called "pain blockers", whereby they would actually perform an epidural on his spine to try to target the pain that he was feeling in his back. The first one did the trick, and it alleviated much of the back pain. However, they had done another only a week prior to the headaches having gotten worse—and, because one of the potential problems with the injections was leakage of spinal fluid, there was a fear that they had somehow nicked his spine during the second epidural. He finally admitted himself into the hospital to try to figure out what was causing these searing headaches.

The doctors began to point fingers, and to disagree with one another about what had brought it on. The neurologist said it was probably the epidural; the pain clinic who had administered the epidural said that it couldn't have been, and that it was probably the cancer traveling to his brain. Yet the MRI didn't show any cancer in his brain. They had done a full-body scan, every test, every blood test known to the medical community, and we were told that nothing had changed. After four days of Colin being drugged to the point of not knowing who he was, they said they had nothing; and that, because the cause could not be found, and the MRI could not confirm whether it was the epidural or not, he would be best suited to our getting another opinion from another set of doctors, which meant another hospital. And so I went to collect him that Sunday and took him home—no better, no worse; just more tired, more spiritually bereft.

He started behaving less like himself; more erratic, more short-tempered. His memory become cloudy and he started to mix up dates, times, kids' names (not just in the shout-out-any-name-that-comes-to-mind way that we all do in the spur of the moment, but completely and utterly losing the ability to recall their names altogether, with the exception of Jake).

Everyone kept telling me at the time how "strong" I was, which only made me feel more guilty and like a fake. I knew that if they could see inside, if they knew what I was really thinking and praying for, they most assuredly would not think that. I was no longer able to see Colin as my best friend, my husband, my whole world. He became the object of all that I felt trapped by. I hated who he had become, and how he had trapped me into this horrible life. I hated the illness growing inside of him, which was in turn becoming the anger growing within me, within our kids, within our family. The guilt was immense—so immense that I hated myself more than anyone else could. I knew the truth about what was in my heart, and I was faking to everyone around me. Everyone was giving their support, their time, opening their checkbooks. I would go to the grocery store and couldn't finish my shop without someone seeing me and ending up in tears. Matthew, who was four at this point, kept asking me, "Mommy, why do you always make people cry? What are you saying to them to make them cry? Why do you make them so unhappy?"

*

Sometimes I still feel guilty, and like a fake. When you are capable of wishing that the person you love would no longer be here, it changes you. I feel guilty about many things I thought and prayed for. At times, it leaves me paralyzed in my own guilt.

*

After that weekend was over, Colin was to return to begin another round of chemo. I had stopped attending every visit. I couldn't deal with the chemo room anymore. I couldn't stand by and watch the poison drain into his veins, hear them ask the same series of questions. I could see that my attitude, my impatience, my hatred of chemo, chemoday; my panic at seeing sick people all around me—people who looked good at the beginning, but were no longer looking so good—it was all forcing me to come to terms with what was going on with us, the fight that we were fighting and beginning to lose.

Colin's brother James, who had always been so good to him, took him downtown on this particular Monday. Colin had his blood drawn and waited for the blood work to clear so he could be approved for chemo. He sat for two hours waiting for the blood work to return, was called in and placed in his chair, and awaited his poison. Finally, I received a phone call from him.

"Jules, they won't let me do chemo today."

"What? Why? It is already one p.m. Did your blood work come back low? What is the problem?"

"They told me that I'm out of the study..." His voice trailed off, like he was falling asleep mid-sentence. Or just didn't have the energy to continue.

"What does that mean? Why on earth are you not getting the chemo?"

"They told me that the cancer has spread to my spine. They discovered it when I was in the hospital, and now they're telling me that I am disqualified from the study."

My heart sank and I felt my empty stomach churning, as if I was going to throw up.

"What does that mean? Why didn't anyone tell us? Why didn't they say anything while we were in the hospital? They said they didn't find anything... what is going on?"

My guilt was now mounting: that I didn't accompany him to chemo, that I wasn't there to plead, to fight, to find out the real answers.

Clearly, he was too tired to fight or understand; too many drugs were building up in his system for him to even care at this point. His will to fight was gone—I heard it in his voice.

"I am just going to come home now. I met another doctor in the hallway this afternoon, who stopped to ask how I was doing. I told him what was going on and he told me to come see him—that he had other studies available that I would be eligible for that have found some success. He told me to go home, to radiate the spot, and then come see him after two weeks."

"Well, that sounds good. We'll talk about it when you get home. Are you feeling okay? What's your take?"

It had been a while since I asked him his opinion: such a very long time since I had consulted him on what he had wanted to do about his own care. From the beginning I had called the shots; I had directed him as to what he should do.

"Well, what can we do? It is what it is. I think he's right. I'm going to take care of the spots on my spine, which may be the cause of my headaches, and then we will figure out what to do from there. I think this is going to be good, Jules, I think this is going to be okay."

"Of course it is, Colin. We'll just have to go back to the drawing board and start over, but it will be good. Just a new start, right?"

I knew that he really had wanted to go see the doctor who had offered his services in the halls of UIC on the way out, but there had to be radiation first and then a couple of weeks for what was known as the "wash period". When you are involved in a research study, the key is to keep all things constant to remove any confounding variables that might be at play. If you aren't getting the results desired in one study and want to join another one, there is a "waiting period", which they call the "wash period"—whereby they wait for any effects from the previous study to surface so that those effects won't taint the proceeding one before you can join another. Although wash periods differ, for Colin it was two weeks. So even if we had found another study to enter, he would have to sit on the sidelines until that period was over. I thought that was the perfect opportunity for us to meet with Dr. Wyatt, a local oncologist I knew of, and attempt to get Colin's pain under control while we waited. We were scheduled immediately for the next day, and again we were off to seek another opinion—another doctor's office, another avenue—when I knew in my heart we were nearing the end.

Before he was kicked from the study, we were on an upswing where we could see the future; our future. Him being released from it was the moment at which I knew, although not wanting to admit it, that the narrative had changed. The problem was that Colin didn't hear it in the same way that I did. Much like the conversation that we had had all of those months before in r. Petty's office about how this was all just a scare, and it surely wasn't real, his interpretation of t being asked to leave the study was "no big deal"—whereas I knew it was quite arguably the biggest deal we'd ever been dealt. When I heard the news, I knew that I not only had to continue to be a fake to my friends and my family, but this was also the pivotal point where I had to begin to be fake with the man I loved the most. His refusal, or perhaps inability, to face what we were facing led me to realize I had to hide my devastation, be his cheerleader, stay positive—be fake. Of all of the things that I have had to swallow, skirt around the issue of, dance away, this was the first time that I felt I was dancing alone. I knew that the cancer had grown to every aspect in my life; including losing the little bit of fight that Colin and I had shared up until this point, to keep him here. He needed to believe he was going to be okay, and I needed to be strong enough to have heavy shoulders and carry on with the charade.

Chapter 20

In the medical field, you hear the word "expert" or "specialist" and you immediately think "this person is someone I need, someone I should listen to, someone who KNOWS better than a regular old medical professional". The problem comes not only when you start believing that is true, but so too when they do. I have seen so many physicians, from every subspecialty, I can't even begin to count. I have also been led to believe that because someone has more education or went to a more prestigious school, or have done things in their past that are commendable, that they get to keep that air regardless of what comes after it. Tayt and Colin have seen the best and the brightest doctors in the world; literally, world-renowned. And so too have they had the misfortune of realizing that, in the end, EVERYONE is human and can only do what is possible. I've talked about the wizard before. Sometimes the wizards you search for aren't the globally accoladed ones. Wizards are found where you would least expect them, doing what you would least expect them to do. How do you spot them? You see it in their compassion, commitment, and empathy. When you get to a point where you understand that someone can't be "fixed" or "cured", you truly appreciate the miraculous nature of some "ordinary" physicians and medical professionals because their care comes from within, not learned in a classroom or from a textbook. I have met many wizards in my lifetime and my loved ones have been blessed by their gifts. They might not have had a cure or been able to make them whole physically, but they have done wondrous things to cure our emotional aches and pains.

*

I woke Colin the next morning to drag him to another doctor. Because this doctor was not well-known, really had nothing to offer that we didn't already know about, and was not in the business of saving "unsaveable" people, I don't think Colin really cared to see him.

We walked into the oncologist's office and waited for Dr. Wyatt. He called us in immediately. I had met his wife at the fundraiser and she had offered his services. He was unlike any of the other oncologists that I had encountered over the prior months. He stood no taller than me, wore an expensive suit and looked very professional, yet also had the appearance of being kind-hearted, empathetic. He wore his feelings on his sleeve, and I think he was completely and utterly shocked at the sight of the two of us. Colin and I had struck a nerve with everyone around us, everyone we touched, everyone who knew our story. We were the average couple: four kids; loving life; involved, engaged, never missing a sporting event; part of the community as best we could be—and now our life was being robbed from us. We represented—to the community, and to this oncologist standing in front of us—not us as people, but the vulnerability that life grants each of us. We all like to live our life feeling mildly in control of the things around us. We all live a life with ups and downs, setbacks, money problems, child behavior problems—and yes, we all have something in our life that is life-altering and all-consuming—but not many people who are just on the cusp of their own adventure, figuring out who they are, starting a family, starting to really enjoy a future, have it taken away—all of it, in an instant. Colin was not in any way at fault for the hand that he had been dealt, and that is the worst kind of illness to be confronted with. You could always feel the uncomfortableness, as if it was contagious; and only until we had left the party, or moved on to another room, did you feel the entire room exhale: as if they were now able to not feel the overwhelming grief or gravity of not only what we were facing, but the fate that any of them could befall. The oncologist's expression was one of sadness, helplessness. It was an understanding of what was still to come, with knowledge of the limited benefit of whatever intervention he had to offer, which he knew would not be adequate.

Although the doctor, who asked that we called him Tommy, was trying his hardest to address Colin, by this time Colin was pretty checked out. He began asking questions that Colin felt unnecessary and a waste of time, and so it was I who answered them. Only when I started to speak of the unceasing pain did Colin start to chime in, to minimize what I was telling Tommy.

After asking me questions and receiving the contradictory history from us, Tommy opened his file to tell us that the cancer had spread to Colin's bones, his spine, and his hip. Up to that point we had heard nothing of the sort. We had gotten bits and pieces from the conversation when he was ejected from the study, but the results of all the testing were never given to us. So as Tommy began to tell us what the results were—himself completely unaware that we had no idea any of this had been found—we sat, staring at him in disbelief, until he looked up from the papers and looked at both of us, puzzled.

"You did know this, right? You knew all this was going on?"

But of course we did not.

Colin finally interrupted him. "So what do we do now?"

"Well," Tommy began, "I know you've said that you would like to continue downtown, and that you need to receive radiation. From the looks of the scan and the results, the areas that the cancer has spread to would benefit from radiation directly at the site. I think that it would grant you a lot of relief. We have a wonderful radiologist that I work with down the hall, and I will call to set it up now. You can probably go straight down there. As far as the pain, we have a wonderful pain specialist within the hospital by the name of Dr. McKay. It seems like you might benefit from a pain blocker like they did to your spine, but maybe if they can target the cancer that is sitting at the base of your spine and shrink it, we can get some of the pain under control."

Tommy came near Colin and asked if it was okay to do a physical exam. I saw the exhaustion on Colin's face. One more person coming at him: listening to his heart (which seemed so stupid, being that it was the only organ that appeared to be functioning correctly), before then moving to his back. Colin winced in pain.

"Colin I really think that you will benefit from all of this, now that the cancer has gotten into your bones." At the sound of that, again a little more of me shattered. "There is a chemo-type infusion that they can give you, which is very effective in stopping the spread of cancer in your bones. I can set up the infusion and if we do it now it should be out of your system in time for the wash period that you need to begin another study downtown." After finishing, Tommy sat silently next to Colin and began to write his recommendations, his scripts. We just sat in silence.

Colin got up from the table once again and began pacing.

"Where is the radiology?" he asked.

"It is right down the hall," Tommy answered.

"Okay, I'm just going to go down there and see when they can get me in."

Like a cornered animal he burst out the door, leaving me sitting in the chair next to Tommy. Part of me wanted to apologize for the aloofness of Colin's behavior, but the other part of me knew that would be a betrayal of what he was going through, and a denial of the fact that Colin had the right at this point to treat anyone and everything any way that he wanted. He had earned that right; and Tommy looked at me as if to say that he understood and that there was no need. He opened the door to the exam room and began escorting me to the front. I realized in that moment that there was no one around. He had cleared his lunch schedule for me; I had not even realized it was lunch, or that people even ate anymore. He walked me to the front counter and told me that he was not going to accept any payment from me, handed me his home cell phone number, and told me to please call him at any time, day or night. I thanked him and walked out the door to find Colin already down the hall, making the appointment with the radiologist to have his hip and spine radiated. It was going to be set up for ten consecutive days for fifteen minutes at a time. The plan was to get the infusion, have the radiation, go through the wash period in which he could have no treatment, and then go back to the University of Chicago to resume working with the head pharmaceutical oncologist who had offered his help to us. I went home, made the appointment with the doctor at UIC, and our new regimen began.

Chapter 21

It has been a long, tough week ... so tough for Colin, well for all of us, but mostly for Colin ... I was commenting the other day to a friend that I feel like our life has become Desperate Housewives or any series that has been on too long, at the beginning it all seemed feasible, yes a little exaggerated, above or beyond the human experience, but still feasible, just intriguing, and then as time goes on and the ratings start slipping, it just gets silly, unimaginable, the writers have to keep upping the insanity, keeping you hooked until you tune in one day and say "that's ridiculous, that can't really happen" ... that is how I feel our lives have been progressing ... I feel as if fate is trying to hold attention by making the story more dramatic to the point of exhaustion and disbelief, so I thank you all for continuing to tune in ... truth be told, I don't have the staying power to continue to watch shows when they get to our point.

Last week three out of four of the kids started school of one sort or another, it is a mixed bag ... nice to have some time, but the silence, the silence has given me a lot of time to think ... sometimes thinking is too much, too overwhelming ... when someone removes the white noise, you notice the deafening of the silence ... that is what I am feeling a loss and a silence without the laughter and chaos of the summer house . . . and am dreading the dreariness of the winter . . . but it's still a way off right? Jake has started his first year at middle school and after going to back to school night at the same middle school I attended more than 20 years ago, I came home full of emotions . . . that was the school where Colin and I carried on carefree, our lives just beginning, freedom just rearing its head and that is where Jake is now, walking the same halls, playing basketball in the same gym, beginning a life of maturity and freedom, he is ready, I am working on it . . . but he is such a cool kid, really, I can say that because I claim no responsibility for it, he was cool from the get-go, hopefully I managed just not to mess with it . . . he is all about the iPod, the cell phone, the internet . . . ugh has middle school changed in most ways, but some remain the same . . . the emotional overwhelmingness of middle school has not changed, the charge in the air is still present, the fear still radiating down the halls . . . I don't worry too much about him, well hopefully not excessively about him . . . I am so proud of him and who he is becoming . . . he is dealing with Colin's illness with such maturity and grace, I am amazed everyday by his spirit and ability to cope . . . at that age, I would have melted away . . .

They began the radiation on the spot of the spine where they found cancer growth last week, and for a day or two, I was seeing some progression . . . I saw for a day or two, Colin resurfacing from the fog he had slipped into for months, the fog that his body had self-imposed to deal with the pain . . . I was so elated to see him get up in the morning, come downstairs, albeit if only for a half hour or so, but that is more than we have witnessed in months . . . yes, I think that I breathed a sigh of do-ability when he resurfaced and I think he actually smiled . . . a genuine smile when watching Pippa, well, be Pippa . . . who we now lovingly nicknamed "monkey toes"... he watched her bounce around the bed and enjoyed having her near instead of shooing her away because she causes too much stimuli to his body that is just focusing on existing in a state of complete agony... I saw a smile and my heart soared... it was working.

We had one good day, one miraculous, elated day, only to be followed the next by the return of the vomiting and a new symptom, an inability to walk... he could no longer move his leg on his own, he had to use his arms to command his right leg to do what his brain was telling it to do. It went on like that for another 2 days until he finally asked them to figure out what now was going on. He had a complete bone scan to find that the cancer has now spread to hip bone, that is why he is having trouble walking, moving, sleeping, breathing... all of it... so now we are radiating the hip bone... trying to stop the spread of it to anywhere else... at times we feel like we are just playing catch-up, it is staying one step ahead of us, while we are trying to reverse it and stay one step ahead of it... after meeting with the oncologist at Good Shepherd, one of the kindest people we have met on this journey, we have decided to try once again the University of Chicago to inquire what trial they may have available... we have been told the standard of treatment, the original chemo, is no longer working, so we need to research something new... we were offered a new drug that has been beneficial on bone cancer which is what it appears we are now dealing with...

My dream now is just peace for Colin, one day of pain management, in his world, there is no such thing... pain management is an oxymoron, non-existent... he finds no relief only in sleep, only in his occasional dreams of a life of no cancer... it's all so unbelievable as I was speaking of before... sometimes the only way that I am able to function *is to imagine that it is not happening at all . . . denial, sometimes is the only way to deal with the situation . . . yes, I am the fortunate one to be in a position to deny its existence at any point of my day . . . my guilt increases as I watch his pain increase . . . when I need to escape, I have some amazing friends willing to drag me from here, help me forget, I thank God for those people every day . . . I don't know how I would survive without them . . . survive is such a funny way to describe it . . . yes, we are all surviving, but we are changing, we are becoming different people, we will never be the same people we were before cancer entered our world, for both good and bad . . . but we have both learned a lot about ourselves in the process . . . so we are back to the drawing board, but have pencils in hand and plenty of erasers to move ahead and be fine with the setbacks . . . we will keep you posted and as always I thank you all so much for your continual support and kind words . . . please don't stop calling, emailing, reaching out, we need you all more now than ever . . . please don't feel like you are bothering us, you are not, you are reminding us that there is life outside of this house, outside of this illness world, outside of this cancer . . . I will try to keep you posted as much as I am able, sometimes we know less than you if you can imagine . . . until next week.*

*

Because of the cancer's having spread to Colin's hip, he was no longer able to move his leg. It was like watching a Vietnam vet who had lost the function of a limb. His mood had improved somewhat—I suppose just because now he knew we had a plan in place, and he once again began to feel like he might be able to stay around, perhaps somewhere inside piquing his desire to fight and be with us forever.

He started coming downstairs for short periods of time. When he saw the children—especially Pippa—downstairs, he'd light up again. The looks on their faces to see Daddy downstairs and a part of their world again was priceless—more than I could have ever given them. He was heavily medicated. He had been given more potent drugs, which made him happy for short bursts of time: able to enjoy being with the kids, and to enjoy laughing and hanging out with them. And for the first time in months, I was able to leave the house for small periods, giving him back the independence he so desperately wanted to exhibit with the kids.

The radiation started to work, and miraculously he began to regain function of his leg. A lot of the pain subsided, and he started to walk and to move again.

After ten days, he was done with the radiation and we were able to just bask in the glory of a small victory. We knew we had a couple of days until we would start back up at the University of Chicago. We had gone to see the doctor in the city. Although he talked a good talk, it all pretty much came down to the same thing that we had heard from others. He had said that, because of the previous trial, Colin was only eligible for two of his studies: both of which showed only minimal results. We settled on taking a drug that had been approved for liver transplants in high dosages, and which was shown to stop the growth of tumors. It wasn't a cure, but the hope was to keep him alive until a cure came along.

When someone you love gets cancer, you become part of a whole world you didn't know existed. Like Harry Potter is a whole world within a world, that is the world of cancer. You begin to find out things that not only did you never know, but you then wish you didn't. Although I understood the importance of a wash period, it did not change the fact that Colin could not start another medicine or clinical trial during that time frame. During that time, every day felt like the cancer cells were growing, one-by-one. I felt as if they were multiplying, gaining strength, making it harder and harder for him to fight against it. I think that there is an impression that cancer treatments have come so far, and made great strides. Every time I turn on the news they have found a new drug to help people survive. Survive for what, though? An extra six weeks? That is what you hear when you actually tune in. They give you the promise that they are moving ahead, but none of the reality. The trials that are running are no cure. And, at a time when you have no time, they require for you to wait for the sake of research. Although I understood the importance, I couldn't help but feel like if they had something, anything, now was the time to give it a try. It wasn't about the greater good for me, it was about losing my husband forever.

Colin really wanted to wait for the study, which sounded mediocre at best, so we waited and we did nothing. The days kept progressing without being able to start, and so did the cancer in the interim. I could almost feel his cancer spreading; and my guilt increasing, at not demanding we do something other than wait. After all those years of making the medical decisions for Taytem, I just didn't have it in me to make any more decisions, especially not when things were calm. Colin was finally hanging out with the kids, joining in with life again, feeling hopeful and part of our world—I couldn't send him back to the thing that appeared to be stealing him away, making him so sick in order to get better. I couldn't force him to do that. Truthfully, I couldn't even suggest it.

All these months later, looking back on the sixteen months that he survived from diagnosis to death, I am forced to see the reality that of course he had some quality time with us. When he was diagnosed I would have given anything for some additional time with him—I thought back then that just any time was what I wanted.

When Taytem was born, I prayed, I cursed, I challenged God that He was not going to take Taytem from me because she was mine: I wanted her here and was not willing to give her up. That was MY selfishness; ME needing her here—I needed her here at any cost. And all those months ago, I needed Colin here as well. I never thought for a minute that he would have to endure the months that came after knowing. Had I comprehended the sheer torture that he would endure, that we would all be forced to endure in watching, I might not have prayed so violently to keep him here. I might have prayed for his peace in passing. Wishes sometimes turn to curses: and as I saw the man I love dwindle, suffer, writhe in pain, turn into someone I didn't recognize, begging me to save him, thinking and believing I could, I understood that what I had wished for and thought I wanted was the very last thing that I could handle.

Although Colin's hip continued to improve, his headaches proceeded to worsen. He was continually holding his head, and had retreated to his room once again. No one was allowed to enter, me included. If I so much as tiptoed over the threshold, yelling would ensue. If he heard one of the kids making noise, he would completely freak out and start crying. Any noise that was made was magnified one hundred percent and was like an ice pick to his brain. I would sneak out with the kids the minute anyone woke, to leave the house for the day: out of fear that someone would speak too loud, someone would make a mad rush for the room, someone would decide they missed Daddy enough to make a break for his room. He would be awake and sleep in the same position. He wore his prescription glasses all day just to watch television; the shades were not allowed to be drawn; the vomiting, which would come on at every meal, was beginning to rot his teeth—his once-perfect smile had turned yellow, and crust was forming in the corners of his mouth from lack of fluids and nutrition.

Colin never considered himself dying; he never let the thought in that he was going to die from the cancer really seep in. There were times when he dabbled with the concept or even questioned it, but his fierce need to stay always overrode his sensibilities about the subject. He stayed in denial, believing that he would fight it at any cost and that he was going to win. Seeing that he was nearing the end, so sick, having so miserable of an existence, I was hesitant to try anything. In my mind, as guilty as it made me feel, I thought that just medicating him enough to get through his days, and to not tinker with anything, was the best way to go about the final days of his life. I had realized that no intervention was going to be successful—it was a no-win situation. If he found a treatment, it was most likely going to make him sicker on a daily basis (like with chemo), or he would find something that would help slightly, but would prolong the agony of what he was experiencing.

However, I would end up going against my better judgment.

When I first learned that Colin had cancer, I feverishly spent the immediate couple of weeks trying to find treatments or clinical trials to save his life. One of the things I came across was the CyberKnife treatment. Colin's tumor had always been most problematic because of its location and size. Since you can't live without a pancreas, removing it surgically was not an option. The CyberKnife is a "surgical" laser that has been useful to cut away tumors of the pancreas when surgical removal is not possible. At the start of my exploration for a cure, however, it would not have been anything that was beneficial or something that could be a "cure", so I dismissed it. Now, though, the radiologist who had treated Colin over the past couple of weeks had brought up the CyberKnife during an appointment with him. Although we were at a point where a cure was not the focus, Dr. Nelson had told us that it could lessen the tumor's size, and perhaps give him some pain relief. Unfortunately, what Colin heard was that it was going to target his tumor—and it gave him hope.

"Hope" is such a trigger word when you are dealing with someone you love having cancer. Hope is good, right? Hope is all that you have; it is what is supposed to lift your spirits, keep you moving forward, and positive. After watching all the suffering that some people go through when they have cancer, hope takes on a different meaning altogether. You no longer hope for a cure. You no longer hope that they beat it. You hope for peace for them. And the absolute worst part is when you realize that the only positive hope you can hang onto is that you hope their suffering ends. That kind of hope isn't something that you feel positive about. It isn't something that you feel good about. It doesn't lighten your spirits, or get you to fight harder: that hope requires that you surrender and give up. For someone who is hoping that the person they love most doesn't suffer anymore, that hope turns into a death wish for them. That hope is the very thing that stings the most, brings on guilt and shame, and makes you question what type of person you are. In the moment, you hope that they will give up and find peace; but, once they are gone, the hope that you had eats away at you. After they are gone you remember the person they were before the suffering, and you then hope that your loved one can forgive you for giving up and ever hoping them and wish that the suffering would stop because the only way it would is if they were no longer alive. Most of all, you hope that at some point you can forgive yourself.

I drove around town, made the phone calls, gathering his latest scans and tests, and made the appointments to meet with the CyberKnife people. After all, how could I deny someone in that condition whatever available treatment that might serve to make his day better? Upon meeting the CyberKnife specialist, we found out that Colin not only had the spots on his spine and on his hip, but that there was more cancer at the base of his brain, right where the central nervous system came in. Months before, that news would have sent me into a panic. Now, though, hearing it came as somewhat of a relief, as we might be able to do something. He said that the other radiologist must have missed it, else decided not to treat it, but, with the great success we were seeing with radiation on the other sites, this might be the perfect solution to try and tame the headaches Colin was experiencing.

In Colin's mind, he was still on the road to recovery; living a long and happy life was still "doable" in his world. He would act like the spread of cancer to a new area was just a minor setback—something that needed to be zapped, and thereafter we would be back on our way to the cure. In my heart, I knew that these "setbacks" were really a road to the inevitable end. I started seeing changes in him that were undeniable. His ability to act like he was on the top of things had vanished. On the rare occasions that he did leave the house, generally just for doctor's appointments, he couldn't even find the energy to acknowledge people. The very few sporting events that he made it to for Jake turned into him chewing gum (as always) and pacing to try to get away from the pain that was coming from within him. He couldn't escape it, no matter how much he ran from it. He was so angry, and rightly so—not only could he not help with coaching, but he couldn't even stand in one place to focus on the game. As he paced, I would watch him pulling up his pants. In the previous two months he had dropped a considerable amount of weight. I felt like I was watching a condemned man walking down death row for the last time. When we returned from the game, he would immediately retreat to his room, out of exhaustion and out of sheer fear as to what was happening to him.

Dr. Steven Nelson was the oncology radiologist we saw. Upon receiving Colin's records, Dr. Nelson immediately got us into his office to begin treatment. By this time, Colin was unable to stand without a cane; and, although his leg was beginning to feel better, there was just something about his hip that was not improving. We sat in the office, waiting on Dr. Nelson: Colin slumped in a wheelchair, me falling all over myself to find something to make him feel better.

After filling out the surveys that preceded every appointment—always the same questions—we were escorted back into Dr. Nelson's office, where we were shown films of what was going on inside Colin.

Although the previous doctor had detected the cancer in Colin's leg, they had mistakenly either missed his hip or were not precise in their treatment of it. In any event, Dr. Nelson came in like Superman and offered Colin the possibility of relief from the pain. Dr. Nelson was very similar to Colin in build, in personality, and in his mannerisms. He was calm, empathetic, soft-spoken, and very positive. He made no mention of the severity or the consequence of what we were witnessing. He only talked about the spot that was missed, and how he could rectify it. As he spoke, I saw relief in Colin's eyes—relief, excitement at being able to change the future, and then anger at the doctor who had missed it to begin with. There was something that he sensed and trusted in Dr. Nelson.

We did what we could to curb the pain and feel as if we weren't sitting around doing nothing. But then, we did have to sit back and do nothing to wait it out. Doing nothing stops you from the very distractions that keep you going.

Those weeks were met with more headaches, and a slow and steady decline of Colin's body and soul—and mine as well. By this time, I had grown tired of talking about it.

After the many trips to the radiologist, there was really not that much improvement. He would have a day where his hip pain would let up, but his back would hurt. Or a day when his back and his hip would give him a break, but then the headaches would kick into high gear. I started saying that every morning his body would have a discussion: "I am tired of hurting", his back would say to his head. "It's your turn; I am going to take a rest, but make sure that you make him miserable—that's our job, you know." Every day I would pray for some peace for him—just a bit of peace. He was losing so much weight that I finally did have to go to the store and buy him some more pajama pants. Not that anyone cared or even saw how he looked, but I couldn't have his pants hanging halfway down to his knees as the reminder that he was not going to recover.

Thanksgiving was coming and he was fading quickly. Before I was with Colin, Halloween had been one of my least favorite times of the year. I hated dressing up: disguising who I was, hiding under makeup, pretending to be that which I wasn't. But there was something in Colin when we began dating that made me love Halloween. He made it seem like so much fun to pretend we were someone or something else in order to entertain other people.

People would always look forward to our big annual party; but here we were—two weeks till Halloween, one year since his diagnosis, and he was down to one hundred and fifty pounds and wasting away. This year there would be no party, and definitely nothing to celebrate. The pain was growing, not getting better, and I couldn't stand to watch it anymore. Finally, I begged him to readmit himself to the hospital. He had maxed out the medications that he could take orally and started to refuse them. He was having a hard time swallowing, and the little appetite he actually did have was being destroyed by the nausea that would follow his taking the pills. And so I convinced him that there was another way.

He therefore finally allowed hospice into our world. The definition of hospice is that you admit that you are not going to receive any further treatment, and it was your last stop before leaving this earth. Of course, I knew what hospice was, but I had no idea that he literally had to say to them—and, more importantly, to himself—"That's it,

I have reached the end of my road and I am ready to go peacefully". Until then we were continually ineligible to receive hospice help, because Colin was always further seeking treatment.

I began to see the toll it was taking on all of us—me, Colin, the kids. The denial over the fact that Colin was going to die was becoming too heavy a weight to bear. Nothing was real. Any conversation we had, anything we talked about: it began to all seem like a lie. The kids had gotten to the point where they were living around him instead of with him. They had learned the drill about how to be quiet, to stay away from his room, to pretend that they didn't see the tears I had tried to hide for so long, but no longer could. It was like we were living in a state of wake, not feeling joy, dismissing happiness because it felt wrong. When we did celebrate anything, there was an instant guilt that we should be relishing in any moments. Grief had taken hold: though we didn't see when it did, we didn't even know that it had. We were too numb to feel much of anything. It was a lie to talk about the future, about treatment, about him regaining any strength, about him rejoining us to live the life we had promised to live together.

I don't remember ever really having a sit-down discussion with the kids about the potential that their father wasn't going to be with us much longer. It was just a quiet understanding that we shared. Pippa and Matthew were really too young to comprehend the gravity of the situation. They never really got to know him enough to know what they were missing, which is incredibly sad to say aloud. Their memories of Colin were more like a sick uncle whom you visited. It was uncomfortable to them; they shied away from a man who they knew as "Dad" but never got to truly know as Dad. Honestly, I wasn't sure what Taytem thought or felt. I always sensed that if anyone could understand what was happening with Colin, it was Taytem. She had lived in the sick world for so long, it was not anything out of the ordinary. Again, how messed up to realize that the most chaotic, heart-wrenching, devastating thing that can happen in families were "nothing out of the ordinary" in ours. Lastly, Jake. We talked around what was happening—almost with a secret alliance, that we were on the same page—but we didn't have to discuss it. If we did, it would almost feel like conspiring. If anyone knew all that we were going to miss, all that was going to be taken from us, Jake did. I believe, however, that he accepted it as I did at some point. He too was exhausted by the dance of "everything is fine, don't look over here". We were both doing it: me for the kids and Colin, Jake for me probably more than for Colin. He was losing his dad, but I believe he was more focused on helping to make sure that he didn't lose me, in the end, too.

It was becoming too difficult to manage Colin's medicines at home. He was never sure when he had taken them, or thrown them up, or skipped a dose and then couldn't get on top of the pain—so I finally convinced him that he needed IV care, which required a nurse. He either had to enter the hospital or we needed to have a nurse in our home: the latter something that we had both dreaded, because it seemed like the beginning of the end.

Hospice had come into my home several times and offered help, as they could provide assistance outside of just medical care for Colin: like grocery shopping, babysitting, everyday chores and obligations. At that time I was completely sinking—drowning, really. I had pretty much isolated myself from the rest of the world. I was running twenty places at once, never doing whatever it was I needed to; and was always paralyzed from fear of something (Pippa overdosing, Colin overdosing). There were appointments for everyone. There were sick kids, there was homework, there was soccer—there was at least one kid needing something every minute of my day. Although I was on autopilot, I was not functioning well. I was angry and resentful. Hospice had offered to help me out with the kids and doing housework. I was reluctant to let them in, as I had always believed that I could do everything on my own. But when it all became too much, I finally agreed to let them in.

The nurse that was going to start working with Colin showed up. I was well versed in nurses, and the whole process was so familiar (the paperwork, the talk about monitoring, the scheduling—by now it was all as routine as breathing to me). The nurse was new; she was a small, Hispanic woman, obviously new to the organization—I could tell by her demeanor. She came to my home and was so well-dressed that I had no idea that she was the nurse. She was quiet and unassuming and spoke very softly when questioning me. The director was with her. Somewhere along the way of the paper-signing and talking and scheduling, she excused herself and asked if it was okay for her to go meet Colin and talk with him. I escorted her upstairs to find Colin in the middle of our room in the small chair, rocking intently.

I introduced them and then made my way back downstairs to finish my conversation with the director. About ten minutes later, the nurse walked down the stairs and sat quietly back at the table. She averted her eyes from mine at every turn—probably no more so than before she had gone upstairs, but, so uncomfortable was she to be around, it was now even more obvious. Soon after she sat down, the meeting was done, and they were on their way out the door, leaving as quietly as they had entered. I got a call from the director the very next day, telling me that the nurse had turned down the case.

"Did I do something? Did we do something? Did Colin say something to her? I don't understand."

There was a long silence on the other end of the phone, as if she was deciding what to say.

"She couldn't handle it . . ." she said, then trailed off.

"Couldn't handle what?"

"Well, don't take this the wrong way—and I know that it is going to sound worse than it is—but she couldn't take the sadness of the case."

"The sadness?" I asked, completely not following where this conversation was going.

"She couldn't stand seeing Colin, so young with four young children and . . . you. She couldn't stand watching what was going on in your home; it was too sad and came too close to home. She didn't think she could handle seeing this case through."

Although I was sad that someone would not take our case, I was not attached to her in any way. I didn't even know her. I suppose, somewhere in the recesses of my mind, I was glad that someone thought my life, our life, so tragic that they wanted nothing to do with it. Her thinking was not unique in that sense. I wanted nothing to do with my own life, and having someone else recognize that somehow made me feel at that moment instantly less alone.

It wasn't until months later, when Colin and I were talking about nothing that was really important, that we were talking about hospice and that first nurse came up again in conversation. I never did tell him why she didn't return. He never asked, and I suppose he never even knew whether she had any intention of returning; we were used to having nurses in and out of our lives. He told me that, as she was approaching him to check his stats—something he was always very reluctant to let anyone do—she inched forward and stepped on his toe. She was wearing high heels, which Colin said literally felt like nails. He had finally let someone come near him, and had gotten stepped on.

"What did you do?" I asked him, smiling.

"Nothing," he answered, and right then I realized that we were both beginning to mellow.

Not give up, or give in—just mellow.

Chapter 21

There are things you admit to others, things you don't, and things you don't even admit to yourself. I now will admit to others that the worst thing that could happen to Colin is not death, when just two weeks ago, I wouldn't admit that to myself. The past month has seen nothing but misery. Colin has remained a tortured soul in his body petering between conscious and unconscious and when the pain becomes unbearable, the subconscious. That is the person that I see most of the time. Colin, my husband, my best friend, he has been gone some time now. The cancer swallowed that complete person months ago, but the essence of who he is, the eyes that I described to you so many chapters ago, those remain.

They are still the eyes of someone who knows too much for his age, those who seem to have a sorrowfulness that burns to his soul. No matter how incoherent he becomes in the midst of it, the pain, the twitching, he will come to life and peer at you with those eyes, and you know that the cancer has eaten his body but his soul remains, screaming out to be saved.

We were ejected from the study when their star patient became their failing baggage without so much as a see you, more with a "and don't come back, we have nothing for you" and he has been playing chase with cancer that has popped up in his spine, his sacral joints, and his hip. He made the decision completely without me to continue on with chemo. A cocktail of poison to stop the growth.

In speaking of what we admit, there were big parts of me that just wished he would give up. Wave the white flag, save himself from the torture, but I understand it. I can't stand to watch it anymore, but when I put myself into his position, I would make the same decision without hesitation. They were offering him nothing more than letting the cancer win, taking the body completely but he loves too much and is not ready to go. He will not give in to this monster. He will not go down without a fight and fighting he is. 150 pounds and in such agony, he can't open his eyes he uttered to me "I am going to beat this," and although I didn't answer him at the time, I thought "if anyone can you can".

I sit here by his bedside filled with so many feelings. I am sure from those closest to me I seem erratic, crazy, perhaps even cold. He has been in the hospital for three days potentially four… Truth be told, I am burnt out, sickened, heart sick. Tired. The last eleven months of Colin's cancer have taken him as a casualty, but he is not the only casualty. My spirit, my children's spirits have been broken, crushed. My children cry for him sometimes and I am torn between feeling so badly when they ask for him and even worse when they don't even notice him gone. He has been a prisoner upstairs in our bedroom for months. It seems every time we fix something, something else falls apart. He had radiation to get the spots on his bones, but then he had blood clots. We have been in and out of the hospital 10 times over the past eight weeks and up until two weeks ago, when I finally cried uncle. I am trying desperately not be angry,

as I said I find myself finding anger, places to place blame on those around me that I have been hurt by in the past. It is almost like padding a Ben. You don't know how to classify the pain and hurt, so you add it onto another service, someone you were hurt by in the past, you add it to their "Ben".

*

I had finally convinced Colin to check himself into the hospital, allow hospice into our home, and start to really get his pain under control.

Him being such an independent soul, that had not been an easy task, and as a result I was left feeling like I hadn't slept in months, walking around in a constant fog. And the truth was, I was falling apart on the inside. Usually you see the crying woman, unable to control her emotions, as the one who is out of control. I was so *in control* on the surface, that it was out of control. I was just existing at best: angry at everyone, feeling abandoned and utterly alone. I was a zombie.

One day when I went to pick Matthew up from preschool, someone called my name. I turned quickly to acknowledge whomever it was, and my foot slipped off the sidewalk. Not my whole foot, just the exterior, which caused my ankle to turn. Then there was a snap. The pain from my foot was nothing—come this point I was unable to feel anything, either physically or mentally. I hobbled inside, picked Matthew up, and exited back out to the car. A crowd was gathered nearby, making sure I was okay, because I had fallen in front of everyone. I made my way to the car, shoved my foot inside, and began to fall apart: screaming, crying, sobbing—not from the pain in my foot, but more because it had opened up something inside me that must have been my emotional floodgate. I sat with my head on the steering wheel, Matthew in the back, wondering what on earth had happened, but not daring to move or make a sound. I finally left the parking lot, knowing full well that this meant just heading home to a life that I no longer wanted to live—now with an added broken ankle. Heading home to a life that I hated more than I had ever hated anything before.

Yes, my ankle was broken. I was on crutches, trying to scurry after Pippa and catch her before she would go to our bedroom and knock for Colin to let her in. Or, more scarily, when she would make it in and then go straight for whatever medicine bottle was open (which usually was all of them). I couldn't keep up. I couldn't breathe. I couldn't go on any longer. The past was catching up with me, and quickly. I was literally falling apart, at a time when I pretty much had burned all my bridges, so my options were pretty limited as far as who to turn to.

Perhaps I hadn't burnt my bridges, as much as I roadblocked them off. I was irritable with people just trying to help, angry really because their suggestions to help made me realize that no one could. The way that they offered up solutions, as if they were really a solution, made me feel as if they thought things were easy or easily taken care of. Nothing was easy. Everything had consequences, or a backlash, or another hiccup or hurdle. And it wasn't just the present situation with Colin's illness. I was burned-out having never recovered from the trauma of Tayt: which I had necessarily shelved, but never packed up and gotten rid of. Most of us have a backpack of past issues that we carry. Mine was becoming a Mack truck that I was lugging around, and I didn't have the strength to pull it along anymore. Yet, I had let go of the people closest to me because it became exhausting to not keep my misery to myself. After all, what I learned a long time ago is that most people are expecting you to say "fine". "How are you?" "Fine." "How are the kids?" "Fine." If you say anything other than that, they are not prepared, and their face usually glosses over—as if they wish they hadn't asked at all. I had begun to understand that either I was placating by covering up how bad things were and living a lie, or I was sick of hearing myself whine, cry, complain. It didn't do any good. Nothing I did seemed to do me any good, Colin any good, the world any good.

When I broke my ankle, it was like I opened Pandora's box. The secret was out; I couldn't go on with the sham any longer. It was a perfect time to let my guard down.

I was no longer able to take care of him, not the way he needed to be taken care of.

That afternoon, I waved it, I waved the white flag.

I had come home, ankle swollen and on crutches, and gone upstairs to tell Colin it was time to take his medication.

"I already took it," was all that he could muster in response.

"When, Col, when did you take it?"

"I took it right after you left to take Matthew to preschool . . ." he said, trailing off.

"But, Colin, I gave it to you not twenty minutes before that . . . you took a double dose?"

As crazy as it was, I hadn't even known what emotions to feel anymore. I felt that, if he was still alive, then no harm done—but I almost wished that harm would have been done. Then instantly, I felt such a wave of guilt that it sent me to my knees. Colin didn't even glance up. He didn't flinch, didn't even notice. I'd sat in that bedroom realizing at that moment that I was indeed utterly alone. Like an actress who is set to go on stage, I looked at myself in the mirror, composed myself, wiped the tears from my eyes, and headed downstairs. In the kitchen I picked up the phone, and finally, after thirty-five years of insisting that I didn't need anyone, I reached out to his parents.

"I broke my ankle; Colin is upstairs, and I can't take care of him anymore. I need your help."

I asked his parents if they could come and get him in the morning and take him to the hospital to try to figure out his pain medications, to get his pain under control. They agreed and I hung up the phone. For the next two hours I sat and just cried silently, not for anyone else's benefit but my own.

Colin's parents collected him the following morning, and took him to the hospital to get his bone infusion. I got a call from him about ten a.m. saying that the infusion was done, but he was going to stop by the house and grab some things because he was going back to the hospital. I felt relieved that his parents had finally been able to talk some sense into him about getting the help he needed.

"That's great, Colin," I said, "I'm so glad that you have finally agreed to let them get your pain under control."

"Well, actually, Jules . . ." He swallowed hard. "I am going to go in and try a round of chemo . . . you know, the one that Tommy suggested."

I was stunned. I had let him go out the door not more than two hours before, thinking that he was just going to try to find some comfort in his world. And, during those two hours, he'd decided to pump more poison into his body. For what? For what end? It wasn't going to make him any better. It wasn't going to heal him, or buy him any time. It was going to rob him of time. Most of all, what it was going to do, really do, the damage it was going to inflict, was hope. Or rather, was just going to give him false hope.

False hope is another kind of ugly that I will never become accustomed to. Most of the time, the procedures that they were suggesting really only came across to him as the cure, the way out. Colin never intended to leave this world. He would endure anything to stay here with us, his family. He would have done anything to watch his children grow. Every time something new was offered to him, what he really heard is that it was not okay for him to go, to leave us, to die.

The hope that I wish he could have been given is the hope that there is something better out there. That there is something beyond this world that was waiting for him, needed him there.

He needed the hope that moving along to another world was what he was meant to do, what would make him happier, make him whole; instead of making him feel that to not try everything—to not try every lifesaving method—would be like him giving up, giving in.

So there it is. The ugly truth. I wonder how many people would "admire my strength" when they know that. No amount of conciliatory tales of "normality" will make me change how I feel inside.

Before we left the hospital for his final brush with chemo, we finally started coming to an agreement about how best to "handle" him. He was growing increasingly frustrated and argumentative. He was belligerent and obstinate: not believing us when we would tell him that he had reached the end of treatment. The doctor had come in and told us that the cancer had reached his brain and there was a huge tumor affecting his eyesight. This was also probably causing most of the headaches that he was experiencing. The doctor felt that the end was near—a week or more, at most. We were being fed all this information, but Colin was not, and so it must have seemed to him that we were all ignoring him. He said to me, numerous times, that I had "given up" on him. I had tried on several occasions to tell him that he was going to die, and soon, but I would look into his eyes and realize that he was not ready to hear it; nor would he believe it coming from me.

As a family we so desperately needed Tommy to step up and be brutally honest with Colin about where Colin was. We needed Tommy to be the cruel bearer of truth. We all needed Tommy to tell Colin that this was the end: that the journey was over, that he was not going to live much longer, that he was done, and he should focus on other things.

We were all seated by Colin's bedside, and the conversation was now slated to take place. Tommy entered the room, and, although we all dreaded the ensuing exchange, we were all anticipating it getting done and therefore none of us needing to do it. None of his loved ones had to appear to be "giving up on him". Tommy sat down next to Colin's bedside, with me on the other side.

"You know, Colin," he started, "that last round of chemo that we just gave you will probably not do much. Our hopes were that it would stave off some of the pain, but it was never an attempt to help out with the cancer itself. There comes a time in treatment when intervention stops being useful and only becomes more hurtful, and you run out of options. And unfortunately, I think that we are there now."

We all sat, motionless, looking at Colin. At this point, we were unsure of what he was understanding, or what he was even listening to.

"So, what you are saying is that I can't do chemo anymore."

"That's right, Colin. Unfortunately, chemo is just not going to help you any longer and might shorten your life."

"Oh," was all that Colin said.

We all sat silently; no one dared to move.

Finally, Colin said "Okay" again.

Tommy slowly stood up and started inching his way towards the door. "If you need anything . . ." his voice softened, ". . . I am always here. You have my cell phone number," he said to us all.

Tommy left the room, and after him followed the other people who had joined in on what felt like a drug intervention, leaving just Colin and I alone in the room.

After about twenty minutes, Colin appeared to almost come to.

"So, I guess chemo's over, huh?"

"Yes, Colin, I suppose it is."

"Well, we better get to work calling those CyberKnife people and Dr. Nelson then."

I sat there, knowing at that moment that Colin would never hear what the truth was. He was never going to come to terms with what was happening, and what was inevitable. Maybe that was the only way that he knew to survive. As much as it frustrated and pained me to go along with it, as his partner in crime I gave in.

"Okay, Colin, but let's get you to your parents' and settled first, and then we'll look for other options."

Looking into those eyes of his—which were pleading me to go along with it, to play the game, to just let him have the fantasy—I had said what he needed to hear, as he did to me about Taytem all those years before.

Colin left that hospital to return to different surroundings. It was so incredibly hard for me to send him to his parents' house; to admit that I couldn't handle it, and that I couldn't take care of him. I felt like I was letting him down, that I had failed him miserably. I was constantly feeling like I was letting everyone down at the same time. His parents had bought a medical bed to put into their living room. The condo that they were renting was a small two-bedroom townhouse in the middle of a subdivision, with very small rooms, but it became the perfect little place for Colin's needs. His parents' house was quiet and tranquil: a much better fit than our home, which was chaotic and overstimulated all the time. They had hired a man to help to take care of him at night. Although Colin was on a pump, he still had to take some oral medications, and he had to push the button on his morphine drip when he needed that extra "oomph".

There were some days when he was feeling especially spry, and on Halloween he decided that he wanted to go to the kids' Halloween parade. All the kids would get dressed up in their costumes and parade around the school. I picked him up from his parents' house, just in time to get Matthew over to preschool and watch the parade. I went into the house to see Colin dressed in his athletic pants, with the fanny pack full of medication tied around his waist. Every time he stood up, that fanny pack would take his pants down. And, because of his delayed (at best) reaction time, he wouldn't get them back up very quickly. We spent quite a while tightening the strap and fixing the pants, but to no avail. Malnutrition and dehydration had taken their toll on him. He had maybe one meal a day that now, which consisted mostly of liquid drunk through a straw because he couldn't see well enough to get the food to his mouth. Most of whatever he was eating would end up all over his shirt instead. He had canker sores in the corner of his lips. When you talked to him it made you thirsty in an unconsciously sympathetic way.

Anyhow, off we went to the preschool: Colin trying to hold a conversation with me and Matthew, but not really making much sense. The first couple of minutes that we were together, he would be completely coherent; but, as time went on, it was almost like he lost the strength or the ability to try anymore, and his voice would become inaudible and his conversation impossible to understand.

We got to the preschool just in time for Matthew to put on his costume and join the parade. All the parents were standing in the courtyard, waiting for their child to be escorted out. Colin began his usual pacing, but with each step he became more unstable. By this time the entire town knew us, knew our story. I noticed that the other parents were looking at him and then quickly looking away, like they were ashamed to have seen what they were seeing. It almost seemed like seeing Colin in that condition was too personal, like something only someone close should watch. No one knew how to react. I didn't know how to react. Sitting in that courtyard, I just wanted to run and hide and say, "Nope, he doesn't belong to me".

The parade lasted what felt like an eternity, after which the children went back to their classrooms. I gathered Matthew as Colin went to sit in the car. He almost passed out when I got in. We were supposed to go on to the elementary school two doors down from our home to attend Taytem's Halloween parade. I asked Colin if he wanted to go back to his parents' house, and he insisted he didn't. I couldn't really argue with him. Realistically, there wasn't enough time to drive him home and then make it back in time to see Tayt. I stopped at home and when Colin saw the house, a glaze came over his eyes and I could see that all he wanted, all he wanted right then in the world, was to go into HIS home and find his way to his own bed to lay down. We left Colin at the house and headed out the door to see Tayt's parade, afraid to leave him there all alone once again. Matthew, Pippa, and I stood on the outskirts of the parade, closer to our home, whereas once I would have been front and center—Colin alongside me, having the flexibility through work to always take the time off. We would have been in the middle of the crowd, talking to others, connecting.

The whole time that I was waiting for Tayt to pass by, I had this feeling of panic inside me. My main goal in all of this was to get Colin back to his parents'. I had finally found some semblance of peace in my life without Colin at home. Knowing that he had found some peace in the confines of his parents' rental home, which felt more like a nursing home, afforded me some time to just exhale. I had experienced some moments of peace for the first time in a very, very long time.

Tayt passed and I quickly began to scamper home, turning every few steps to ask Matthew to walk faster. I needed to get Colin "home", and I needed to get him there now. I left Pippa and Matthew in the kitchen and walked upstairs to see Colin in his regular position—head propped up, pillow under his knees, all color drained from his face. At this point he was on so much pain medication that when he slept, he appeared to be dead. It was so shocking and it used to turn my stomach, and I would walk into the room loudly in order to try to get him to wake up before I could see him looking that way. Knowing this, as I neared the room, before I got to the doorway, I called ahead,

"Colin . . . it's time to go, you have to take your medication."

"Okay," was all he said. He fumbled, trying hard to sit up without assistance yet unable to, until I helped him up. "I can't sleep here tonight?"

"No, sorry, Colin, we didn't bring your medicine, you have to go back to your parents' tonight. Maybe another night . . . I know, maybe I will ask my mother to take the kids for an overnight so that you can come home and spend a night in your own bed. That way they won't keep you up. Would you like that?"

We made our way downstairs, put the kids in the car, and headed back to his parents' house. I was so thankful at that point to have the excuse of his missing medication. That meant there was no question as to whether he could stay. It was not simply me telling him he could not sleep in his own bed that night. The guilt of telling someone you love and who is dying that they can't have something as simple as sleeping in their own bed is overwhelming, something I can't describe. He was never to sleep in his own room again—in our bed. It had become my bed.

An entire year had passed since his diagnosis, and true to his prediction he was alive. Not really living, but he was alive. Jake's birthday was coming, and Colin wanted to make sure he would be there to celebrate. All Jake wanted was to bring the DVD of his best football game this year for Colin to see. So we picked up the DVD and went to visit Colin. The plan was to get dinner and bring it back to his parents' to eat. Colin decided for some reason that he wanted to go to Red Robin for dinner, so off we went. The ride was almost perfect—Jake in the backseat, Colin talking to him about the sports radio that was on until we finally turned into the parking lot. Colin told me to pull over, so I pulled into a space immediately and he proceeded to throw up several times. I repeatedly checked on Jake in the backseat, my heart so heavy that this was his birthday "celebration", and here we were, stuck in a car, listening to Colin vomiting. I didn't know whether I should just stick it out or turn the car around and go home. No one was hungry anymore. There was tons of silence. Finally, Colin said to us to go on inside and he would come in, asking me to leave the keys.

"Remember," I said, "you are not allowed to drive."

He looked at me as if he wouldn't even consider it, so I left them on the seat. Jake and I went into the restaurant and sat in the entryway, waiting, looking out the window and watching the car lights blinking over and again. I kept watching Colin in the car, finally realizing that he was in the driver's seat.

"Are you sure you don't want to go out there?" Jake kept saying.

Finally, I saw the car reverse. I ran outside to see Colin driving the car around the parking lot—the wrong way. It was as if Matthew had stolen the keys and was taking the car for a joyride. I ran after Colin.

"Where are you going?!" I screamed. "Park the car! Pull over!" I was yelling at the top of my lungs, terrified that some child would dart out into the parking lot and Colin wouldn't have the reflexes to stop fast enough, nor the forethought. He finally pulled into a space, and got out of the car like an old drunk: stumbling, and saying something about, "If you would just stop yelling at me . . ."

We did end up eating before heading home. After a long silence on the drive back, Jake and I started recalling what had seemed like a horrible situation—and, you know what? We started laughing . . . we were able to replay the entire scene back to each other, finding humor in it.

We laughed all the way home. Not in a "making fun" way, just in a "Colin is still in there" way.

Chapter 22

So, yes, Colin is now staying with his parents. His treatment ended four weeks ago and when the headaches wouldn't stop, being here was too much for him, the kids, the chaos, the noise. He ended up hiding up in our room, literally didn't come down for 12 weeks, like a prisoner, I brought him meals and cleaned up his dirty plates... I couldn't stand to think that he would live out the rest of his life locked in a bedroom, hiding from all of us and me, carrying on life as if he were already gone because I couldn't stand the guilt of not being able to coax him out of there. So, I have begun a mental list of all the things that I miss about Colin. Yes, I know he is still here, but there are so many things that I have begun to notice that he is to me... so many things that I took for granted, things he did, things he took care of, things that seemed alright because he made them so... the list is overwhelming and debilitating if I let it overcome. Most of all, I miss Colin's smile and his honesty. I realized the other day that it has been months since I have seen him smile, a true, happy life-affirming smile has not crossed his face in so long I have started forgetting what it looks like. You think that you will never forget, but you do, you do so quickly... so quickly. I am fighting daily to remember Colin as he was a year ago, not as we are fighting this illness now, but the full of life man that is my husband. Colin had asked that I bring over our wedding pictures three weeks ago, so last week, I woke up in a panic at 3 am, I ransacked our basement looking in bins upon bins (some of them I am convinced are filled with rock), to find our wedding pictures hidden at the back of the closet, of course at the bottom . . . It was such a mixed bag to look through them, it seems like a lifetime ago, we will be celebrating our 10th wedding anniversary this year . . . it just doesn't seem like enough time.

The kids have really started missing Colin, especially Matthew. The other day I was sneaking downstairs to get something from the kitchen and was just passing the stair landing when Matthew came bounding out of his room screaming "Daddy?" . . . It was as if he thought Santa was here . . . you could've ripped my heart out and I don't think that it would have hurt that badly. Pippa, my crazy child, when we visit Colin crawls up in his lap and just calmly hugs him and lays her head on his side . . . for once, she maintains calm . . . they all voice how much they miss him in the oddest of times when the house is quiet and you think that they aren't thinking about anything in particular . . . it is very confusing to them that Daddy is sick and is not getting better . . . Matthew is constantly and obsessively asking me "what happens if you get sick?" and then runs through the list of the people he cares about "and Nana, and Grandma", making a mental list of all the people he can potentially lose . . . it really does break my heart.

As for Colin, he has his good days and his bad, oh . . . I am so lying, he has his bad days and his God awful . . . every day brings on a new torture whether it is vomiting, headaches, it just never seems to let up or give him a day of solace, but he keeps forging forward, talking about getting better, when he gets better and we all keep praying that he knows something that we don't and that the doctors are wrong . . . I just pray that he will stop suffering so immensely . . . it is literally taking my soul a little more every day. He has stopped answering his phone as he did . . . but he does read his emails when he can manage to focus his eyes, so please don't think your messages have gone unread, and please keep them coming to him . . . he needs to know that life has not left him behind . . . and me, well I suppose I have stopped answering my phone as well. I noticed the other day that my phone had not rang in a while, I had not gone out in a long time, talked, laughed . . . I am either home with the kids or over with Colin, I haven't even been shopping in months trivial I know. I am having a hard time coping with the reality of what is happening, watching Colin suffer, being stuck in this roller coaster that was never fun, but completely devastatingly torturous now . . . and yes, I feel like life has left me behind. I worry that there will not be a day that we will smile and laugh again . . . not like the laughter that Jake and I shared, the laughter to break the emotional breakdown that we are feeling, but true laughter, unencumbered . . . the kind of laughter that hurts and makes you cry at the same time, I worry that we will not ever do that again . . . and mostly I am missing my best friend with all of my heart. There is nothing worse than going over to visit Colin and realizing that the things that we used to talk about, to share are of no concern to Colin anymore . . . it all seems so trivial, I feel like I have lost my whole world. But I have these wonderful, fun, energetic, beautiful children that pull me from the depths and make me realize that life will and has to go on, because they need me . . . and certainly more than I want to admit, I need them.

So we are taking it day by day literally day by day, we try not think about things too hard, just trying to get through the day . . . but it does feel like we are on an island sometimes . . . I watch television and feel like the whole world is spinning and we are standing still, never changing . . . it's so hard to be stuck in a position of such grief, stress, emotional discord . . . I think it has robbed us all of perspective, maybe that is good, maybe that is the only way that we can survive this, if that is what we are doing . . . yes, that is what we are doing, surviving.

*

Seeing Colin alert was hit or miss. It depended on the day, the hour. Diana would give me updates when I would call, but in order to really believe what she was describing you would have to witness it. You see, Colin was always able to "pull it together" when I was around: to not hallucinate, not talk to objects that were not there, not to be belligerent or mean. For me he was always able to be Colin, at least for the majority of the time. People would come visit Colin: which was far and in between, and mostly on his insistence. He believed that he needed to instead save the time: to get better, and for his family. He felt that having idle conversation with someone was robbing him of energy and time, so he refused most visitors who wanted to come by. The few people who did come to visit, always relayed the same message. I would hear their conversations and it would always end with "keep fighting, Colin" or "hang in there, Colin". The message was always that he should continue to fight, that dying would be like giving up, that choosing to move along was a bad thing. I think we do and say things like that because we think that is what they need to hear, but I began to sense that Colin needed something different. He needed someone to tell him that it was okay for him to go. I think that he needed me to be that vehicle for him. Any chance I had, I began whispering in his ear that it was okay to go. Whether he was awake or asleep made no difference—I knew he heard me.

I used to say things to him like, "Colin, it is not giving up. There are better things ahead for you. Don't keep fighting to stay here. Your body is done; there is only misery left. We will be alright, Colin. I swear we will be alright. Take care of yourself; find some peace."

Whether he was sleeping or not, he would sometimes appear not to hear me. Most of the time, though, he would just look at me, confused, and ask, "Where are we going? Why do you keep telling me to let go?"

But I persisted. I felt like he needed me to forge on.

I was beginning to let only my close friends into my real feelings—my wanting him to go, my need to move on, my need to not see him suffering continually. I couldn't bear any of it any longer, and I was really starting to crack. One of my friends dropped off a book to me after hearing me talk about trying to get him to move on: one, written by hospice nurses, about how people have to finish business here before they feel alright about moving on. I began to try to think of what Colin could possibly need to hear in order to move on, to let go of his hold here on earth—and, perhaps selfishly or self-servingly, I thought that maybe his tie to me was what was keeping him here. All the time that we were together, I rarely told him how incredibly much I loved him. I was never the touchy-feely type, and to put myself out there on a continual basis scared me to no end. So, although our undying love was understood between the two of us, I thought that maybe he needed to hear me say it, really say it. I resolved to let him know: to free him of worry about us, about what was going to happen to us when he finally let go.

The next day, when I went to visit him at his parents' house, I waited patiently for them to give us some time alone. I sat there, just waiting for the right time (if there ever was one), to really let him know all that I wanted and needed to tell him, in order to set him free from any unresolved feelings he might have had. His parents finally headed upstairs. Since Colin was tired, he asked if I would help him lay his bed down. I of course did, and when I finally felt that the room was quiet, I began to speak. He was lying all the way back: eyes closed, hands folded in front of him. I wasn't sure if he was asleep or not, but I was bound and determined to say what I needed to say, thinking that, surely, he would hear me somewhere in the recesses of his mind.

As I began, the words came cautiously and softly.

"Colin, I just want you to know that although I'm not very good at letting you know how I feel, you are everything to me. I can't remember a time when you were not in my life. Everything we have been through, you have been by my side, holding me up. I couldn't have made it this far without you. I don't know how I am going to go on without you."

At this point I was literally choking on my words; unable to breathe, yet trying so hard to continue.

"I love you more than I have ever loved anyone, or will in the future. You were my first kiss, my first love, my forever love. I just love you so much . . ."

I choked out, tears flying as I was letting it all go. All the emotions I felt and had held inside, afraid to put myself out there: I now decided, there and then, that I would not let him leave this earth without letting him know all that he meant to me.

"I am so, so sorry if I haven't been there for you . . . I promise that I will take care of the kids, Colin, I promise to love and take care of them. You don't need to worry about me or about them. We will all take care of each other. It's time for you to go, move on, be free."

Tears were streaming. I saw that Colin was beginning to stir, and then it appeared as if he was trying to get up.

"What is it, Colin, what is it? Do you need something?"

Wiping the tears from my eyes, I almost thought he was going to sit up to talk to me.

"It's just that your crying is bugging the shit out of me . . ." was all that he said.

I helped him sit up a bit, then turned, grabbed my things, and headed out the door.

I was angry and frustrated. That was so Colin: to negate what I was saying. It was too much, too intense for how he was feeling—so he shut me out. But I know he heard me. I know deep down he heard me. Whether it set him free or not, it set me free. The other part of me felt relieved to know that the Colin that I loved—the feisty, sarcastic Colin that I loved—had not yet left.

The estimated two-day time limit that he was given turned to days, then eventually to weeks, then to months. It was almost like watching a horror movie: you would think surely he was at his end, but the next day he would be coherent and fighting harder than before. He never stopped asking when we were going to seek other opinions. I didn't know what to say when he kept asking for doctors. He would go on these rants: insisting that he needed to see an eye doctor because he couldn't see. At first, I went through the whole explanation about his brain tumor and how it was pressing on his optical nerve. He would look at me sadly, and quietly say "Oh", and then it would be over. He would forget about it until the next day.

The headaches were becoming unbearable, not only for him but for all of us. He could no longer really see at all, and had fashioned a makeshift eyepatch. There were times when he covered the one eye that he could see better out of. It was obvious that he would be better off just shutting his eyes while talking with us, but he had already lost so much of his world. Being able to be present and see around was one thing that he was not going to give up. One day, Colin was really at his wits' end. His headaches had increased at a rate that was uncontrollable. It was hard to distinguish what was physical pain and what was mental anguish—or whether there was a difference in the two at all. The social worker, the doctor, Helen the nurse, Diana, Ben, Colin, and I were all sitting in a tiny space discussing what we were going to do to help him. At a certain point, Colin couldn't take the meeting anymore and just got up and left the room. I went to find him. It was a two-story condo and he was hiding on the staircase. He sat at the bottom of the stairs, attempting to get away from the discussion of his situation.

"Colin, what's wrong? Are you alright?" I asked when approaching him.

He was sitting on the stairs, head in his hands, with just one tear in his eye. He looked up at me, eyes out of focus.

"Why aren't we seeing doctors, Jules? Why don't they care? I keep asking to see doctors and no one is listening—no one hears me."

"You want to see doctors, Colin? You really want to see doctors? Who do you want to see? I will call and make an appointment. If you want we will get you to the doctors . . . is that what you want?"

"Yes," he said, and put his head back in his hands.

I got up from the stairs and headed back into the other room, returning to the meeting with a new objective.

"All right, I just spoke to Colin and he would like to see a doctor."

They all looked at me like I was out of my mind.

"He just needs to see a doctor," I asserted. "That is all that he wants, and it is making him miserable that when he asks it is falling on deaf ears. He's lost all control over his life, and every time he asks for a doctor we all just change the subject like he is two and will forget. He is not forgetting And I think possibly the lack of control and the frustration may be contributing to the headaches that he is describing. I know he is not well—probably not well enough to make it to the doctors—but he is miserable. And if that is what he wants at this point, let's make it happen."

I knew at the time it was not a solution. It was not good for anyone involved. But Colin needed it. He needed it, and I needed to make it happen for him. There were not many things, if any, that I could do to help him, to help take the burden away—and if this was the one thing that he wanted, then I was going to make it happen.

After the room cleared, I called Dr. Nelson, the only doctor that Colin would feel satisfied with seeing. I thought surely if he saw Dr. Nelson, the doctor could talk some sense into Colin and make him see that he needed to stop searching for answers and treatments that were not available anywhere. I made an appointment and the very next day Colin and his parents were on their way to another radiology consultation. I was unable to go, as I had been neglecting just about everything at home and it was all falling apart. Thanksgiving was coming, and life was getting crazy with school parties and events; the kids needed me too. I knew that whatever was going to go on in that appointment was purely between Dr. Nelson and Colin, and I almost considered it better if I stayed away. Later I got a phone call from Colin. He sounded tired, but very upbeat.

"Hey, Jules, Dr. Nelson thinks that they can radiate the spot on my brain and make my vision better."

"What? He thinks that you should go for more radiation?" I asked in disbelief.

"Yeah, he thinks that it would help out."

I started getting very panicky. They had talked about radiating the spot so many months ago when he was in the hospital, but the consensus was that the risks of doing so—mainly frying the brain tissue—did not warrant trying it.

"Are you sure, Colin? Is that what your parents heard? Are you planning on doing this?"

"I don't know, Jules; if you want you can call him." He barely had enough energy to finish the call.

"All right, Colin. I will come to your parents' later to see you."

When I hung up the phone I instantly became enraged. I couldn't believe that any doctor could see the condition that Colin was in and suggest that he go for further treatment. I don't know what scared me more: that they would radiate the spot on his brain and he would be a vegetable for whatever time he had left, or that its success would ultimately prolong his agony. I was afraid that doing something like this just meant a longer time to stay on this earth and suffer.

I picked up the phone and dialed Dr. Nelson's number. He was the kind of doctor who actually answered his own phone. I was a little unprepared when he picked up the phone on the second ring.

"Dr. Nelson," he said.

"Hello, Dr. Nelson, this is Julie Barth, Colin's wife . . ." And then I paused, trying to collect my thoughts and decide the best way to approach this situation without sounding insane and selfish and crazed. "Colin told me that you told him he could do radiation on the spot on his brain?"

"Yes, I believe that if we do a couple of treatments of radiation it may alleviate the pressure on the back of the brain."

"I don't understand—we had discussed radiating the brain several weeks ago, and were told that it would be too risky and that there was the potential of killing the brain tissue?"

"In my opinion," he began, "the tumor is in a place where it could be radiated effectively and safely, and might give him some relief from the headaches—"

At this point, I was highly frustrated and angry, so I cut him off.

"I think," I began, "that it's become pretty apparent that the headaches are not coming from the tumor at the base of the brain. He had these headaches months ago—in fact, almost a year ago—and they had nothing to do with the brain tumor. He didn't have the brain tumor back then, and still had the headaches. It is beginning to look like the headaches are coming from the mental anguish of what he is struggling with more than anything physical. In my estimation, by giving him the notion that something can be done to make him better you have just further given him more to anguish over, more hope—that is the reason why he refuses to stop fighting and let go."

"I'm sorry that you feel that way, Mrs. Barth. I lost a very good friend about six months ago to cancer myself—young, like Colin, with very young children—so my heart goes out to you. I am so very sorry and I never meant to make things worse. I was just thinking that maybe we could help make his pain a little less. I will let him know that it is not a good risk to take; I was just hoping to reduce his headaches."

At this point I felt awful. I began to think that I didn't want this for Colin because it would prolong my agony—not his, mine.

"I don't know. I just don't know what to do or think anymore. I just want him to not suffer anymore. I just want it to be over for all of us."

Colin called later that day to let me know he had spoken to Dr. Nelson again, and that the doctor had changed his mind and believed that radiation was not a good idea after all. Colin sounded deflated, but more exhausted than anything else. I believe that, somewhere inside, he was relieved. Like me, he had given it one last attempt at not going down without a fight—but he didn't have to try anymore; he could rest, and let whatever happened happen.

I decided that, for Thanksgiving, we would just have a small lunch with Colin at his parents', and then the kids and I would have an equally small dinner at our home later on. I felt like the kids needed to have a quiet dinner, something really low-key. I believed that was all any of us could handle at the time. However, we showed up at Ben and Diana's around noon to find that the entire family was over there. Both of Colin's brothers and their families had come by to visit him, never mentioning this to me beforehand. When we showed up it seemed like a three-ring circus, way out of control. They were going to head to Diana's sister's house after this.

The trip to Diana's sister Dory's was literally only five minutes, but the ride there was miserable. The motion of the car would start off Colin's vomiting, which by now was never much more than dry heaving (he had nothing left in his stomach). His eyesight had gotten so bad that he couldn't see his hand to get it to his mouth properly, so he was unable to feed himself. The majority of his calories had become liquids fed via a straw, or an occasional ice cream bar; and anyway, whatever it was would end up finding its way back out an hour or two later. He made me pull over two times on the short ride to dry heave. I was so angry—so incredibly beside myself—about how his family was so unaware of what they put him through by showing up to have a party next to him, and then making him feel obligated to leave the only comfort he had now: the safety of his "home". When we arrived at Dory's, I went around to his side of the car to assist him with getting out. He didn't want my help: so it would consist of several pushes with the elbow to indicate that I should let him be, followed by the stumbling, and then submission when he realized that he had to let me help or else he was not going to get there. We walked into the front door and I quickly found a spot for Colin to sit and set up camp. He tried to eat something, which only ended up being thrown back up, leaving me to clean it up. After about forty-five minutes of doing nothing, he looked at me and said he was ready to go. That was the last Thanksgiving that we shared. I dropped him off at his parents' and went back to pick up the kids. They had already eaten in my absence, and were not happy that I was pulling them out early.

Two days after that was Colin's birthday, so the kids decided that they wanted to have a party for him at Ben and Diana's. After the fiasco of Thanksgiving, I was reluctant to have all the kids packed into that small a space for any length of time. But, it was really important to them. So we picked up dinner and brought it over to their house. Jake and Colin were hanging out, watching football in the living room (which was now Colin's bedroom); Tayt and Matthew were playing in the front room; Pippa, who was completely out of control, was running around like a madwoman. It was nearly half-six in the evening, which was very close to her bedtime, and we were all waiting patiently for dinner—all except Pippa. She became unruly and obnoxious, and the more tired she became the worse it got. Knowing this about her, I started seeing signs that "crazy Pippa" was about to emerge, so I tried to hasten things up a bit. We all sat down to dinner on a long table in the middle of the room and ate macaroni and cheese and hamburgers. Colin had about a bite and then was finished. We had some cake, then clean-up began.

As dinner had progressed, Colin had decided that he wanted to say something to all of us. He shushed everyone and started:

"Thanks, everyone, for coming here to celebrate Thanksgiving with me."

No one corrected him. The kids didn't even notice—it had become the new normal to just overlook the fact that most of the time Colin was completely unaware of anything that was going on around him, nor had any concept of time. Pippa was sitting on a barstool next to the kitchen table, waiting for cake. Then she dove straight over the side of the table, missed, and landed headfirst on the floor. When I say "headfirst", I mean her chin hit first and then I heard the most unearthly noise—it was a *crack*, like a bone breaking. I ran over, scooped her up, and stood her on her feet. She was looking at me stunned, not even crying. I stood in front of her and tried to get her to stand. She was still looking at me, but looking more *through* me, and every last ounce of blood had left her face and body She looked like she was going to collapse, and was having a hard time standing. I quickly gathered everyone together and got into the car to drive home. On the way home, I asked Jake,

"What do you think, Jake? Do you think I should take her to the emergency room?"

"She did hit pretty hard, and she doesn't look so good," was his reply. "I can watch Tayt and Matthew if you want to go."

I thought about it for a minute, and knew in my heart that if I did not go and have someone tell me she was going to be alright then I would worry about it all night. After four hours of waiting and a five-minute conversation with the emergency room doctor, it was determined that she was fine, and we returned home.

The days dragged on. Every one was the same. I would go to his parents' about mid-morning and visit with him while he fiddled with things, slept, and talked in his sleep. He no longer had the wherewithal to pull it together when I would come visit. I still let Jake go whenever he wanted (Colin would have had him move in if Jake wished.) Every time I saw him the deterioration was apparent to everyone, and it became painful to even be around him.

About two weeks before Christmas, I had a great idea to call his parents and see if they could bring him over so that we could all decorate the Christmas tree as a family—perhaps for the last time. The day before I arranged it, he had seemed to be having a good day, and so I thought maybe just for an hour or two he might be able to pull it off and create some final memories.

I remember at the time wishing at this point that he at least waited until after Christmas to die. I was so afraid that if he died at or around Christmas, that that would forever be the memory that would haunt our children at a time that is normally so joyous.

His parents agreed to bring him by, and just about an hour after the kids got home from school, Colin was dropped off at our doorstep. He came into the house and I noticed that just the fifteen-minute trip from the condo to our house had drained him more than I would have thought possible. He was shaky, grabbing his head, looking for a place to find solace in the chaotic home that used to be his. He entered the back room where the Christmas tree stood and sat down in our oversized chair, immediately grabbing his head. Knowing this was a very bad idea, but completely lost as to what to do about it, I gave all the children ornaments. I kept handing these to them to place on the tree: as a distraction for them, and to keep them away from Colin, who obviously could not take the strain that this visit had placed upon his already failing body. As I was having Matthew put one of the last ornaments on the tree, Pippa noticed for the first time that Colin was sitting in the chair. She made a beeline right for him.

She jumped straight into his lap. Not knowing what was going on, I heard the most horrible cry come from Colin's direction, and looked over to see Colin doubled over, Pippa standing next to him in tears. I also noticed that the pain medication line that was supposed to be continuously administered had been knocked out. I panicked. I grabbed the phone and began dialing Ben, who had literally just dropped him off. Pippa knocking out his IV meant that they would have to call hospice and wait for them to come hook it back up again. Diana told me that Ben would be on his way, not indicating if he had yet made it home or not.

I hung up the phone, once again feeling like a failure. Again, I had tried to create something that I knew wasn't to be. I just wanted—needed—so badly to make everything okay. As a wife and as a mother and as a woman, you do everything in your power to make everything okay for the ones you love. I had had seven years of trying desperately to make everything okay, to exert some control over what was going on in my life. All to no avail. I had failed at every junction: and this night, and the memories created during the tree decorating, were no different. The kids have long since forgotten, but I have yet to forgive myself for those moments when I couldn't just leave well enough alone.

Christmas was upon us. The kids had been out of school a week already, and apart from maybe one family visit, they had been entertained by other things, away from the sadness and despair of the condo. On Christmas Eve, I called Ben and Diana's to see what plans, if any, they had for the day, and what exactly I should do with the kids and Colin. We decided I should take the kids to their house, open a couple of gifts, decorate their version of the Charlie Brown Christmas Tree, and spend some time there. Colin was having a really, really bad day, so I knew realistically we would probably only stay a short while at best. His headaches and vision problems and mental state had deteriorated to the point where I was wondering how much of "him" was really in there.

Colin came into the room as the children were playing, and sat down next to them on a fainting couch.

"I want you all to know . . ." he began slowly and deliberately, "how grateful I am that you all came. I want you to know that I love you all truly so much, with every part of my heart, and I am so proud of you all."

With that, Pippa started toward him. Cringing, I tried to intercept her, but Colin held out his arms to her and for a brief moment he was the strong, loving, powerful Colin that he used to be. She ran to him and he scooped her up into his arms. Tayt and Matthew saw this and realized that it was alright to touch him for the first time in a very long time, and they ran to his side as well. They did a group hug, the kind I thought would never end, and when they emerged there was not a dry eye in the room.

"I want you all to go home now and enjoy the day. I also want you to go to bed tonight on time, so you don't miss Santa Claus."

I was astonished. Colin had not been able to form enough of a thought to recognize one of his best friends two days before, but now he was coherent and loving and was the Colin and Dad that we all so desperately needed. He had given us all the greatest gift possible. That last Christmas, he gave us the gift of seeing the person we craved for one last time. He gave us the gift of seeing the person he used to be; the person who was still inside; the person we all missed so very, very much. We went home, had a quiet dinner, never discussed the morning's events, and watched a movie together (which we all dropped off during). I then carried everyone except for Jake up to bed, after which him and I played Santa Claus: wrapping, eating cookies and carrots, placing the surprises under the tree. Jake had taken the role of Colin in these few short months, and I don't know if I would have survived the time without him. He was only twelve, but behaved with a maturity I have never seen someone his age be able to muster.

The following day, Colin was not well enough for us to see him, so we spent it opening and playing with gifts. I don't know what I found to be more profoundly sad: that Colin was not there, or that no one really noticed. We all carried on as if there was nothing missing. We were all beginning to live life without him.

Chapter 23

I got the same call I get daily today. "Colin is asking for you, you better come." Tayt pretended to be sick today to take the day off of school, and the car is in the shop, so of course, called my mom again. I took my time getting here as I usually do, made the beds, cleaned the rooms "why are you doing this" I question my mind . . . the answer comes in the same every time. "Well if I have to be there a long time, I don't have to worry about what is going on at home."

*

"What's up, Colin? What's going on?"

"I am in so much pain, Jules, so much pa—" This was cut off by a wave of pain that went over him and stole his breath and his words away. "Come put your hands on my head." I instantly realized he wanted me to do this because he knows my hands are ice-cold. The room was so electrified and so intense that I couldn't do anything but stand paralyzed.

"Dr. Rose is on his way," I heard Ben say. "He is coming, Colin."

"Is he going to give me a shot to put me out of my pain?"

"Yes, Colin, I am sure he will have a shot."

Like waiting for an ambulance, every second turned to agony; one minute turned to a thousand. "Colin, he is coming; he will make you feel better."

I was afraid these were his last moments and had things that I wanted to say, but I felt the pressure of the people around me to not say what I really wanted. I wanted to tell him to go. I wanted to tell him that it was time to be free, to not be afraid—the words I'd uttered to him hundreds of times over the past fourteen weeks. But this time I wanted him to hear me and listen to me.

I heard the door open and close, and realized that his brother had come in. He stood there, looking at me as I was sitting on the bed next to Colin, holding his hand, silently crying, ready to explode with my thoughts and words.

"I am so sick, Jules," Colin began, and then crying—although no tears would come because he was so dehydrated.

"Think of something else, Colin. Try not to think of the pain. Think of our wedding." And then, in the madness of all of his pain, he chanted under his breath: "I love you, I love you, I love you" about a hundred times.

I didn't know if he was imagining our wedding, or just wanted to make sure that I heard him. A lot of what he said in those days fell upon deaf ears—he didn't have the strength or the infliction in his voice for anyone to hear it—but it was important, it was always important.

"Think of when Jake was born," I said.

I just kept throwing out scenarios for him to think about, which made my tears come even harder.

"I can't do this anymore, Jules. I can't live like this anymore. I don't want to be here."

For the first time, he had finally started raising the white flag.

"I know, Col. It has been far, far too long."

The four people hovering, waiting on the magician to come and take the pain away, finally saw the doctor pull up to the curb. Colin continued to writhe in pain.

"I don't understand," he continued. "I just want to not be in pain, I want to d—" before trailing off once again.

He had started to talk some gibberish about his parents not being able to take care of him, about how we hadn't made the right medical decisions for him, and how Ben should be able to fix his eyes.

Colin's stepfather feels things like no other human being I have met. He loved Colin with his very soul, not that we all didn't, but Ben agonized over Colin's every wish. Whatever it was that Col wanted, Ben wanted to be able to produce. He had become Colin's "fix-it" man. He had caught the mistakes in medications that nurses had been unable to, had become Colin's personal masseuse, he had done it all (along with Colin's mother; but in a much different, almost indescribable way).

Two days before, Colin had had Ben in tears. As I say, in Colin's hallucinatory world, Ben could fix his glasses. In his world, Ben could take them over to the kitchen, grind them, pound them, and make Colin see again. Ben's heart broke that he couldn't do that for Colin. It was killing him that he couldn't do anything for Colin.

Upon his arrival Dr. Rose quickly went into action, changing the IV drip—doubling it, giving Colin ever-higher dosages. I had the thought that this must have been how Colin had felt, sitting by my side as I gave birth all those times. The doctor left to go into the other room and the entire family assembled in the kitchen. The wagons were circling and all I could feel was more tension and apprehension in the air. I was summoned to the kitchen where the doctor said, "I can give him 5mg of methadone, or I can give him ten. I know ten might be a lot, so I can start at five. He shouldn't have any problem with the ten, but if you—"

I stopped him mid-sentence.

"Give him as much as you can. Don't jerk around with the five; just give him ten." I returned to Colin's side, and he looked up at me: the months of torture showing in his face. His eyes, unable to focus, were pointed in different directions, and his mouth was contorted in the most unnatural position: as if he could not control even the very movements needed to speak.

"Jules, it didn't work . . . none of it. It didn't work; I am still in pain, I'm still dying; it didn't work." I gently sat down next to him. "I know, Col. You're right; it didn't work out the way that we planned. But do you remember when Taytem was born? It wasn't what we had wanted. But look at the beauty of what we got out of that situation. If Taytem has taught us one thing it's that sometimes we don't get what we want. And sometimes the things that we do get look horrible and terrible at the start, and it takes getting beyond them to see the beauty in it. If Tayt has taught us any lesson, that is the one I carry with me. It is that sometimes you just don't get what you want. We have no control over the hand that we are dealt, but in the end it always works out. You just have to get beyond it to see it . . . you just need to get beyond it, Colin . . . do you understand me? This body is done; you can't stay here. I want you here more than anything in the world, but you can't stay. You need to let go; you need to find some peace."

He closed his eyes partially, as if to shut me out. From that point on, he went through periods of time where he trembled, and when he looked as if he wanted to say something, but his mouth wasn't allowing the words to form. Those were the very last coherent words that he uttered to me, and in turn the very last words I am sure that he heard. From that moment on, he slipped into a permanent state of hallucination. At the time, I didn't know if it was the high dosage of narcotics that had been administered, or if we were really facing the end. He started having periods where his hands and feet were ice-cold; but this would be fleeting, and within minutes the warmth would return and the chill traveled somewhere else. The doctor told us that it was the body's way of getting ready to go. He told me that, at the very end, that is what happened: parts of the body, circulation, management would completely shut off. He was getting ready to move on, his soul was beginning to find its way out. Although there was a part of me that was looking forward to Colin being out of pain, there were so many parts of me that were not ready to let go. To this day I have such a feeling of despair that I was capable of wishing him gone. I just can't find a way to forgive myself.

He spent the day making gestures with his hands, talking to and yelling at objects we couldn't see. I don't know if he was hallucinating or talking to spirits, but it almost looked like he was telling whoever it was, "I'm not going; do what you want; I am not going to go with you". At times he would gesture in the air, like he was crossing things off his list. Other times he would be giving the high-five sign to some imaginary guest. The day was filled with so much activity it was tiring to watch—tiring to see that he was still searching, still trying to act out whatever was in his mind. He wasn't trying to find peace, but to reconcile something in this world, something within his own mind. There are the ever-present whispers, everyone is trying to keep the noise level down, everyone wants to be quiet. It reminded me as I sat there of when I was a child and I attended a funeral. We have all been in the funeral home when the whispers overpower the quiet. Those whispers, when placed together, add up to be quite a loud symphony. That was what it was like there—a funeral parlor, twenty-four-seven. The tiny whispers, the skirting around, the muffled thoughts.

When you are in crisis mode, an hour can pass by in a minute and before long you realize that you have lost days, even months. That day seemed like an eternity in some respects; but, when the sun fell, it felt like I had just gotten there. Finally, the majority of people had left. Some would come in and it would become uncomfortable, and then they would say goodbye, kiss Colin, and scoot out the very loud door. Colin, who had been silent most of the afternoon, had started to become more anxious. For anyone who has watched what I prayed to be the last days, even hours of someone's life, it is torturous when some begin what is termed "terminal delirium". (Not be to confused with plain old "delirium" evidently, and I am assuming it was a phrase coined at some conference to "ease the death process in".) As the darkness grew and the time advanced, we would all pace in and out of the room: grabbing his hand, and all saying the same phrases, as if programmed—much the same way men do when coaching football or watching a game ("choke up", "that was a pick"). I don't think those phrases are taught, they are part of our human spirit. "It's okay Colin, I'm here Colin, you are okay Colin": those phrases just come off of the tip of the tongue even more unintentionally than when you kiss a baby—most of the time completely unaware that you are even doing it, to the point you would fight someone who called you on it because you genuinely don't remember it.

As night fell, Diana, James, and I were left in the room. I had always known that my mother-in-law was a beautiful woman—that was always evident. The way that she carried herself, there was just something about her: an eloquence, a mystique that was lost somewhere in the past. She had an aura about her that was indescribable, magical. She sat in a fainting couch: very, very tired. This road had not been easy on any of us, but much more so Ben and Diana. Diana, going through chemo herself, was still carrying on, staying up all night, worrying the worry that only a mother can feel. Since her ovarian cancer diagnosis nearly twenty years earlier, the cancer would return again and again. The way that she stayed on top of it was by measuring her blood levels. The minute that they would spike, she would begin chemo again until things normalized. At any given time, she was either back on a chemo regimen or waiting to be back on it again. I always saw her inner beauty, though, and when she sank into that chair, I began to think if I had not met her as "Colin's mother", I would have seen the extreme beauty that she had on the outside (just as how you can never see your own mother as being attractive). She sat back with such elegance, and her face almost came alive when she talked about Colin and the "old house" and the mischief that the boys used to get into.

The younger Diana came out. Not the tired, cancer-fighting, a-mother-worrying Diana, but the young, innocent, fun Diana. I was able to see her for the first time as a person; someone that I liked not just because I had to, but someone whose company I was truly enjoying. We sat in that room: her reminiscing, laughing, talking about the trouble that Colin used to cause. Stories of the time he tried his stand-up comedy routine that, being far too raunchy and obscene, was booed off of stage (mind you, the entire family was there watching, never expecting that language or those topics to be discussed by Colin). It had been completely out of character—but that is what had made it such a lasting, funny memory. The ease of the conversation returned, and we sat like we would on the screened-in porch all those years before, when Colin and I would hang out and drink with Ben and Diana. The insults, real or imagined, of so many years had disappeared, and we were just old friends getting together and talking.

As the night progressed I sat at Colin's side. His unceasing hand gestures, his working through his time here on earth, never stopped: that he was trying to justify it, to finish whatever was keeping him here, was apparent in his hallucinatory actions. James went home and Diana, already shot from the day, had excused herself and headed upstairs, leaving just Ben and I alone with Colin—my Colin, who looked more like an air traffic controller. The doctor, who had initially stuck around to make sure that Colin was no longer crying out in pain, had left as well, and so the condo was quiet. Ben and I were pretty much pretending out of necessity that the other was not there. Ben, who had been with Colin since he was two, really was Colin's dad more than any natural father could be, sat down next to Colin on the full-sized bed that they had moved into the living room. Colin had felt the medical bed to be too hard, too cold, and had resorted to trying to climb upstairs to be in a bed that was more like home. And, after a couple slips on the stairs, and Ben and Diana finding themselves unable to help him up and down them anymore, they had the night nurse help them move the full bed downstairs to make Colin more comfortable, and he had immediately made it his permanent bed. Ben got into the bed and laid down next to Colin, whispering things to him to try to comfort him. Tears were welling in Ben's eyes, and I looked away to give him the time he needed to resolve what was going on in that room—that Colin might be physically still breathing, but he was gone and not coming back. It got very late, and although I didn't want Ben to have to stay with Colin all night by himself, I also knew that I had not been home all day. The kids were worried, and were now probably all asleep besides Jake, which made led me to be afraid that Jake would be up alone, worrying about Colin, not knowing what was going on or why I was not home. And I knew that the next day was going to be a tough one. The doctor had told me that Colin would not make it through the night, and if he did, he most certainly wouldn't make it through the next day.

I looked to Ben, my eyes so tired and dehydrated they were stuck open, and told him I was sorry but that I needed to go home. Truth be told, I needed to spend the night in our bed. Not my bed, but the bed that Colin and I slept in throughout our marriage. I needed to feel connected to him: not the Colin that was hallucinating in front of me, but the Colin that I had spent the last eighteen years with. I needed to find some familiarity, some comfort, some safety—if only for a brief time—in a room that I thought I could never feel safe in again.

I got in the car. The weather was rough: the temperature outside had hit an all-time low, and being just a couple days after the new year the snow was piled high and the roads icy. I drove quickly, much too quickly for the conditions, just needing to be in the safety of my own home.

When I returned, the house was quiet because everyone was asleep. I crawled into bed, not bothering to remove my clothes, afraid that I would get a call in the middle of the night to come back. It felt so wrong to even try to get a couple of hours of sleep, but as soon as my head hit my pillow I drifted off. I awoke a couple of hours later, jumped out of bed, and headed straight back to the condo. I had overslept a bit and, although I was there early, it didn't feel early enough.

I took a seat right next to Colin and saw that he had not stopped his hallucinatory movements. Ben indicated that these had continued all through the night. Ben looked exhausted, and although he was always able to just go along through Colin's illness (and likewise, the many years that he lived through Diana's illness), the ordeal was beginning to take its toll. When I finally looked at Ben—I mean really looked at him—he looked like he had aged years in just the time I had slept at home. I took a seat down next to Colin and watched as his brothers and his aunt made their way into the house. There was a constant shifting of people from one room to the next as I sat by Colin's side: constantly whispering to him; constantly reassuring him that it was time, it was time for him to move on. Although he never acknowledged, I knew Colin well enough to know that somewhere, somewhere deep inside, he was still there. That he could hear me, and he was listening.

I reached over to feel that Colin's limbs had all gone ice-cold, and his breathing and hallucinatory movements began to slow. He was no longer moving with fluidity: he was moving slowly, as if winding down. His limbs were no longer listening to whatever his brain was asking them to do. I inched closer and his breath began to slow. Noticing the quiet, his aunt and his brother entered the room and found me sitting by his side. I had moved from my chair onto the bed to hold his hand. He began to gasp, trying desperately to take air in. You could feel the panic in his body. He didn't say anything or open his eyes, but you could feel through his nonverbal communication the terror that he was experiencing at what his body was doing. His mind had not yet come to that conclusion, but his body was done.

Colin's aunt began to chant Hail Mary over and over, telling Colin to look for Mary and to look for Grandma, to not be afraid, to go. I wanted to say something to him, but I was embarrassed, or maybe just stunned at what was going on. I didn't know what to say, afraid to voice it out loud in front of other people. But I finally stopped worrying about what I was saying and who could hear. It was the most intimate moment, and although it felt wrong to share that moment with anyone besides just Colin, I no longer cared who heard me.

"It's okay, Colin, it's okay. It's time to go. I love you more than life and I am going to miss you more than I have words. I need you here, but I need you to move on more. Your body is done; it can't be here anymore; you can't stay anymore. Don't be afraid; please, Colin, don't be afraid; where you are going is beautiful and wonderful; it's a place with no pain, no illness. I will come with you, Colin; we will never be without each other. You go ahead, you set up camp, and I will meet you. You have to go ahead, but I promise I will meet you, and I will love you forever. Don't be afraid; go ahead and get it all set for me".

His breath began to come in short bursts, then started to come minutes apart. It was completely surreal. Although I knew it was going to happen, I was not prepared for watching those last breaths leaving his body as they were. He was not fighting anymore, and I began to wonder where he was going. If there is ever a moment that makes you wonder about what happens after you die, then sitting that room, watching him take his last breaths here on earth, shook my belief system, making me wonder where you go, where was he going. His soul left without any notice. It left without any form. It was so unbelievable, and to this day makes me question existence—what happens, and where it is the soul goes. I suppose someday I will find out.

I stood holding his hand as his last breaths were taken, whispering to him to not be afraid, to go ahead, to wait for me, that I would love him forever.

All at once, I recognized that he was gone.

My Colin, my love, my husband was gone; he had moved on; he was finally free.

I let go of his hand and sat back on the chair by the bedside. I remember people scurrying around outside of the room, doing things, moving, hugging . . . I don't remember anyone crying or showing emotion. The hospice people had shown up for the end of it, and had gotten busy disposing of his medications; there was a mad rush to count and flush. I began to realize that I needed out of there. I didn't want to commiserate with anyone. I didn't want to stay, hug, comfort. I sat down next to Colin in the room that no one dared to come back into, and I put my head in my hands.

Colin was gone—he was finally gone, which left me with a sinking feeling that I had to go home. I had to go home and see my children. I had to tell them that their father was dead. How on earth was I going to get through that? Sure, they knew he was dying, but how was I going to be able to tell them that he was gone, and they would never see him again? I just stood there for what felt like hours: trying to gather myself, trying to get it together enough to head home, to tell them, to let them know what had just happened. I got up quickly, resolved to head home and let them know, and as I moved around the bed to grab my bag, I mistakenly hit his foot. In a knee-jerk reaction I turned to his body and began apologizing—"Oh my God Colin, I am so sorry . . ."—before trailing off. It was such an immediate reaction. For months, if I had hit his foot like that it would have caused him misery, the slightest tap enough to summon tears. But here he was: I looked to him and realized that, for the first time in fifteen months, he was no longer in pain. I no longer needed to say I was sorry for living, for moving, for being around him, for touching him. He was finally free from pain, and I was finally free from watching it. As sad as I was that I had lost the person I loved more than life itself, I was happy—I was elated that I no longer was able to hurt him mistakenly, that he was no longer able to be hurt at all. In that moment, it was such a strange feeling to be elated. But I was. And then, just as quickly, the guilt returned.

Chapter 24

I had known for so long that it was going to end this way. Not only had I known, but I felt I had wished for this very moment: for Colin to be free of the body that was continually failing him; and, to be honest, for me to be free. See, it didn't matter where I was. When I was with him, I felt guilty to leave the kids. When with the kids, I felt guilty to leave him. And always, always, I felt guilty that potentially the very last place I wanted to be was at his side. There can't be any worse feeling than to want to make things better for the people that you love. To sit and watch as their very soul is taken from them, not ripped from them, but just broken off continually in pieces. That is how it felt, that is how I felt for years at a time, forced to witness as my loved ones disintegrated in front of me. Watching from the sidelines, knowing that in my heart I would have traded his life for my own. That is not a saying, it is true there was not a turn along the way that I would surely not have given my life to not have to be party to the pain of spectator. I would have substituted my very own body to not have to feel so utterly useless and paralyzed. I had people begging me, believing in me, believing that I could do something to make them better, to make them whole, to make them something other than in misery, but in the end I could do nothing. I know that at some point there needs to be a way that I can forgive myself for my actions, for my thoughts, for the way I felt, the things I wished, prayed and hoped for, but that day has not come. I am completely incapable of forgiving myself or thinking that I deserve anything but misery. Misery is what I live and misery is what I believe I deserve.

*

So many months later—as I sat in my kitchen on a Sunday morning: making pancakes, music playing, all the kids up at the bar waiting patiently, talking amongst themselves—I began to feel something. Something that I hadn't known I was missing, or perhaps something I never aspired to feel again. I felt the faintest tinge of happiness well up in me, the tiniest piece of hope. The very hope I was so upset that Colin had had, and here I was experiencing it. It was foreign to me, and in an instant I felt two things that overtook the feelings of happiness: guilt, and terror. I feel guilty all the time to have survived; and like, if I were to survive and be happy, that would be a betrayal of Colin. And if by chance I were actually to be happy, sheer terror would follow knowing in that instant that happiness is so fleeting, so unpredictable, so fragile, if I were to feel happy, it could all be ripped away again, all the things that I love, all the things that I have, ripped away from me in an instant. It has happened before and I am afraid it will happen again. My smile and happiness fades quickly and I continue on my day, with guilt in my heart and a pain that just wanted cease.

*

I walked in the door at home to find that everyone was there. The house was in utter chaos—not the bad kind, but the kind that it was always in, with kids running everywhere. I felt a heaviness in my heart: the dread of telling these four young children—who worshipped their father, who loved him with all their hearts—that they would never see or talk to him again. Even through the confusion and the illness, it was Colin they wanted. It was their dad. Sick or not, they loved him so thoroughly and with all that they were. Even if he yelled at them, or called them by the wrong name, or was angered easily and often, he was just Daddy to them, and could do no wrong. Here I was, realizing that whatever I would say to them in the following moments would be forever marked on their soul. Whatever words or phrases I uttered were not going to be inconsequential to them, or something that they would lose: they would be burned into the psyche as a moment in time never to be forgotten, probably to be lived time and again.

"Hey guys," I said, trying to crack a smile. It was an odd feeling: as if I almost knew a secret that I was about to share with them. Yet most secrets are happy, most secrets are the kind that you have to hold yourself back from sharing. This secret, the secret of knowing that Colin was gone, was one I wished that I could take to my own grave. "Matthew, where is everyone?"

"I don't know, Mommy."

"I want you to be a big boy and get everyone together. I want everyone to meet up in my bedroom. I have something that we all need to talk about."

I don't even know why I chose that location. Our bedroom had become the worst place that I could think to inhabit—maybe that was why it was the first place I thought of? The grief that I was about to disseminate felt like the plague, and I wanted to keep it just for us—us five, grieving alone, without any interruptions. It was just us five against the world now.

Matthew did exactly as he was told, and had everyone gathered in the room.

Pippa—who was barely able to talk in full sentences, though who sensed there was something in my eyes and my demeanor that needed protection and her extension of love—met me at the entrance to the room to take my hand. We guided each other toward the bed, where everyone had assembled. I stood at the foot of the bed, speechless. All the things that I thought would be so important to say, the things I had considered, the things that I had practiced on the short ride over—gone. They all escaped me. Here I sat, staring into the faces of my children who needed for me to be strong and to show them that it was all going to be okay, and I just collapsed. I bent down to pick Pippa up and set her right down next to me. I wanted to reach out to each of them and hold them all as I said the words that almost felt like betrayal:

"Your daddy went up to heaven, guys," I said in nothing more than a whisper. I was looking down when I said it, but quickly raised my eyes to see them all looking at me. There was nothing in their eyes that I had expected. There were no tears, no anger—just an understanding; maybe a pity for me that it was stripping all that I was to say it to them. Of course, they were too young to understand the gravity of what I was telling them, but I had practiced the inevitability of what I was going to say with them, almost as a fire drill; maybe all the practice had numbed them to what the words actually meant. I looked at Jake.

He was looking at me with such astonishment. It wasn't like he didn't believe, or was not expecting this moment to come, but more like he wanted to save me. He looked at me like he just wanted to take the pain and hurt from my eyes and make me okay. He then scanned the room, looking at his siblings and determining how everyone else was handling what I had to say. Seeing that they were not fazed, he looked back again, searching: searching my eyes to find me in them, knowing that I was not present in what was going on.

I had checked out; I had numbed myself to what was occurring. After about two minutes, we all leaned in to hold each other. I can't remember how long we all sat there. No tears were shed; no one cried out, or questioned. There was a silent resolve, knowing that we would make it through all of this. There were events and things to come, but we would all get through it together. It really was the five of us against the world.

Chapter 25

Much like a lawyer works on their summation, I will write this, rewrite this, start over, mull over every word, every thought, every phrase that is written, and in the end, I will read it and see it's imperfection because I know that there are no words afforded in the human language to describe the feelings and thoughts that are in my heart and my very soul. Yesterday the world lost a soul: that of a human being who was wonderful both inside and out. Colin was not ready to leave this world, nor were we ready to let him go. To the very end he fought to stay here: not for himself (nothing he ever did was for himself), but he fought because he knew we will always need him here. His very last conversations, being barely able to speak, were filled with angst of not being able to help, not being able to "do"—never the utterances of the "unfairness" of what was being done to him, never the selfness of what he was going through: just the sadness of not being able to help us all. Peace came over him, and when he finally realized that to go would not be to "give up", he allowed himself to trust in God, and follow the path that was laid before him. He understood that whatever God had planned for him was greater than anything that he had planned for himself. After he was gone, I sat at his bedside, not crying because he was no longer here, but because he was gone. I sat in tears wondering what I could possibly tell our children that would make it acceptable, understandable, the least damaging, and I knew, knew for certain that whatever it was, they would be able to see through the facade to know that I myself didn't understand why he had to leave us, what was calling him away from us. As I turned to leave, I grabbed my jacket and accidentally hit his foot. "oh my God Colin, I . . ." forgetting much as you do when you pick up the phone to call a love one long since gone on auto pilot, I was jumping to apologize, already sick to my stomach instantly, because that is the suffering he was enduring the past couple of weeks, the slightest movement, the softest sound became unbearably hurtful and pain searing. I looked over to find that he wasn't wincing, writhing in pain from my touch. He was at peace, finally, I saw a body that was no longer suffering and in a way that your humanity feels is wrong, but your common sense knows right, I was happy that he had moved along.

I came home to gather the kids and walked into a home somehow changed and in other ways not changed at all. Matthew and Pippa were eating and I summoned them all upstairs. We all walked to Colin and my bedroom, the bedroom that we shared for over 10 years, I sat them down, took a deep breath, fear in every morsel of my being, realizing that these young souls are looking to me, solely to me to give them guidance when I am so uncertain myself in my own future "your father went to live in heaven today, Daddy died today", I felt I had to say "die" in order for the gravity of the situation to somehow stick. As I looked into their eyes, into the faces, my fears began to dissipate . . . I looked to each of them to see within their hearts that Colin was not gone. He had given not only life to these three souls, but he has given them wings, and confidence and love and life lessons, albeit learned to young, but ones that will give them the ability to fly and fly they shall. It was sitting there, looking into their faces that I realized that within each of them Colin carries on to spread the goodness that was Colin, the kindness, the incredible giving that Colin possessed.

During one of our very last conversations, Colin was in such excruciating pain, he turned to me and said "it didn't work Jules, it didn't work, I am here in pain, it wasn't supposed to be like this, this is not what I wanted"... his voice barely audible to speak "you are right Colin, this is not what either of us had planned, but do you remember when we had Taytem? That was not what we had wanted either, she was not what we had planned. The lesson that we both learned from Taytem is that sometimes we don't get what we want, and what we get appears to be horrible, terrible, unimaginable looking from it where you stand. But when you get beyond it, you are able to see the miracle in it. Taytem was our miracle, and if there is one lesson that we learned from her is that there are better things ahead"... he closed his eyes at that moment and silence fell upon the day. It was at that time that I realized that the senselessness of what Colin has been going through, what he has endured, if we don't all recognize it, it will not have the full potentiality that it was meant to have on us all. I know there will be some that will have regrets about the past year, you are not isolated, you are not alone, we all have the regret of not being able to do something, we all wanted to be able to do something, but please know that there was not a moment, a single moment along this journey that Colin did not feel loved and supported by each and every one of us. I believe that Colin came here for a specific reason and lived his life to the highest degree of the lessons that he taught us all. There is not a soul who is not better for having known him. There was a point in his illness where he was so worried about the children. He was worried that they would look back and feel as if he abandoned them, that he didn't fight hard enough to stay, there was so much pain in his eyes as he told me this fear. "Col, you have given your children a gift that most people will spend a lifetime trying to give . . . . a love to them, as well as me, that most people will search their lives to find . . . they will know of your courage, your undying want to be here, to fight, to stay. They have learned about perseverance, compassion, selflessness . . . those are the things that they will remember, those are the gifts that you gave to each of them. In your short time here, you have taught them lessons of a lifetime that albeit too young, they have learned and will carry on to teach all they touch."

*

So, yesterday we all lost a husband, a father, a son, a brother and a friend that will be truly missed beyond, well beyond words. So as we are all devastated, at a loss, lost, we must remember that to not continue to live on to laugh, to love . . . would be a disservice. Colin asked of me one thing "Julie, promise me . . ." and his voice trailed off, I was so fearful that he would not continue with his wish and after a long, thoughtful pause he said "joke". I knew what he was saying, he was asking to not lose our sense of humor, to always live life to the fullest, joke about the things that are the hardest and look at every challenge with courage and humility. He wanted us all to continue to live each moment to the fullest, enjoy, please enjoy the time that we have here, because it is fleeting, it is spontaneous, miraculous and for anyone who knew Colin, it was so damn fun! He loved his life tremendously, he loved his friends, he loved his family... he loved life. Colin gave us all wings so that we may fly, he gave to us gifts that can only be repaid by sharing them with those around us. He will be missed beyond words... truly beyond words... So please hug your spouses a little longer today, hug your children a little tighter, and try to hold onto the fragility you feel about life at this very moment, because it is fleeting and fragile, but beautiful and elegant and enjoyable to the highest degree... to the very highest degree.

*

When the funeral was over, I packed—if you can call it that—and haphazardly (at best) threw the kids and odds and ends into the car, and we began our journey to Florida to find some warmth, and subconsciously to find some pieces of Colin left at the very place that I remember him smiling. On the beach. Asking me to take a picture. Talking about a future for him—for us. I needed to close his life.

Jake knows about this book. I told him as a pipe dream that this book will keep us housed and will bring to us the prosperity of kings. I know it's not true, but I need something hopeful to hold onto. I need to believe that the fates that stole my best friend and the life that I had made for myself can now deliver great things. I know in my heart they will deliver compensatory things at best, but I needed to feed myself and Jake a fairytale. I needed that fairy tale because otherwise I couldn't carry on or to live this life that was in shambles around me.

Jake asked me where the story ends. I don't know what to tell him. "When I have said everything that I need to say, when our new lives begin, that's when the story will end." The truth is that, if that were the case, then this is it—this is the end of the story.

My story, Colin's and my story, it ended the day I saw him take his last breath; arms folded across his chest, gasping: first for air, and then calm coming over him with peace of some sort. Not the peace I had expected, not relief, just acceptance that it was the end.

So off we headed on our journey. I needed to find security, to find safe. I felt like I was a victim of a violent crime, and I was—a crime of incomprehensible magnitude. Someone came in, they tore my world apart, they killed my very best friend, the person I love most in the world, and—to add the highest of insult to injury—I had to watch it in a slow, meticulous, incremental, torturous way rob us of his life, his smile, his faculties, his very existence, even down to the memories that I have. It robbed even the memories I hold.

*

As I watch the reel of any memory as a film in my mind, at the end there is that "in loving memory" line tagged to remind me that what I was watching was the last, the very last of the happy memories for Colin and I. Because no others can be duplicated, cut down, reproduced again. Those are the only memories that exist, and I know they will never be again.

They have robbed me of him forever. I will never be able to laugh with him, joke with him, tell him I love him. I know that our love story has not ended, we will meet again wherever he is waiting for me. I know he is waiting for me somewhere, and I fully intend to join him again and pick up where we left off, but I miss him with the most heaviest of hearts and although I have these beautiful children who force me to carry on, I would, if given the option, throw in the towel and go join him now. But now, is not my time. I do find some comfort in those final hours for myself when he will show himself to me, come to take me with him, and that is a time when my heart will heal and soar and smile again.

Saying Goodbye—My Eulogy

"As I was trying to find something to wear to mass, I said to one of my friends, 'I don't know what to wear. I don't know anyone whose husband has died so young.' And it's true. I could find it easy to fall apart and feel sorry for myself, to ask 'Why me?' But then I realized that it was not about me. The person that I admired most in the world—the person who was my world; the person I said I would spend the rest of my life with—that's who this was about. Colin gave of himself even when there was nothing more he could give. He was devastated: not that he was sick, but that he couldn't give to us anymore. For those many months, as he suffered indescribable pain, he did so in silence. He never wanted to bother anyone; he never wanted anyone to pity him or do for him; he wanted to do for himself and not put the burden on anyone else. Colin was the bravest soul I have ever known or will have the opportunity to know in this lifetime. He loved life with a ferocity that captivated everyone around. He had the ability to engage you, make you laugh, get you excited, make you believe in things that you'd thought not possible. If Colin said he was going to do something, it would be done. He was an optimist to the highest degree, and believed in those around him, in me, in those dark times when you no longer believe in yourself. He was patient and kind to everyone he knew and believed in the dignity of the human soul. I used to get so jealous of Colin's ability to make our children laugh, at the fun that he would bring out in each of them. The happiest part of the day was when Daddy would come home. They would all run to the door to greet him. I don't know whose smile was greater, his or theirs. Children loved Colin. I always believed that it because children could see his good nature feel his warmth, know the goodness that he possessed; his honesty, his openness, loyalty. His stay on this earth was far too short, but he taught me lessons that I could have lived a lifetime without learning. He gave me the friendship and the love story that people spend their lives searching for. So, I don't feel sorry for myself. In fact, I consider myself one of the luckiest people alive to have had the opportunity to have him in my world for the time I did. I will miss him, a little more every day—the memories of his illness fading, to give way to the person he was: the person so full of life, vibrant, happy, living life to the fullest.

Truth be told, I have not yet begun to miss him. It doesn't seem real. It doesn't seem possible that this person, so endeared by so many people, is not here with us anymore. I will feel his loss for eternity, almost as if my right arm is missing, but I know that Colin would want us all to carry on: to continue to laugh, to love, to smile, and to find humor even in the unfunny things. For he knew that, once you were unable to find the humor in things, life was no longer worth living. Right before he left, I said to him that we would all see him in heaven. I told him to go ahead, set up camp, wait for me, and that we would be together again. He had the strength to begin that journey ahead of me, and I know he will be waiting with a smile on his face and his arms stretched wide when we meet again.

For him and I, for all of us, the best is yet to come."

I awoke this morning in and out of sleep it has been three months since Colin has passed on in a way it seems like years ago funny how when your entire life changes you get so used to the change that you forget what you used to be like, what your life was before, you get glimpses, but think "that couldn't have been me". I was dreaming that Colin's family and I were at a summer party. I was juggling kids and heading to the pool, but for some reason I had forgotten my swimsuit (sounds right). So I was sending the kids with his brother, and my friend Anne handed me the keys to his car so that I could run home. From the corner of my eye, I saw Colin's stepfather sitting on a bench, looking like he was in pain. I walked over and his stepfather said to me, "I have this pain right here" as he signaled toward his neck. I hesitated. Most of the time when people find out that I am a fitness trainer, they tell me all their muscular issues, so I was ready to give him my analysis of what had happened; for some reason, I remained silent and reached out toward his neck. When I touched it he made a noise that indicated he was receiving relief while being in pain. As I rubbed it more I could feel the knot, and I said to him, "That's it, I found the knot. I know it hurts, but if I can work it out, it won't hurt anymore." Then he turned to me and I finally saw that it wasn't Ben—it was Colin. His soulful eyes, the ones that I have fought desperately to put out of my mind, stared at me as if to say, yes, it's me, I am here. I woke up with a start, tears streaming from my eyes. Him being there felt so real that I was able to reach out and touch him one more time, but I awoke to find myself alone, unable to reach him again, almost like starting all over.

So it's been over a year—fourteen months to be exact—since Colin's passing. So much has happened, although it feels like it was just yesterday. I find myself getting lost in my day, not realizing that something has changed, then I look around and find that everything has changed; nothing is the same. I've pushed back tears for so long, it is as if they have forgotten how to fall. They are mixed in with every emotion I feel, only I don't know they are there. They're tossed around inside, and it only makes the emotion more murky, yet doesn't overtake the entirety of the feelings themselves. At times I miss him so immensely that I feel myself spinning in circles when I realize that for a brief second not only is he gone, but that he was ever with me. The smile that I see in his pictures: that's what I fight to keep foremost in my mind, instead of the images of his body, so riddled with cancer. His once-immense body, decreased to weightlessness. His mind, that was once so quick and witty, reduced to talk of insanity. Seeing faces that were not around. Seeing things that did not exist. I was the one person he always felt could save him, but this, the one thing that he really needed me to save him from, I couldn't. I couldn't ever make it go away for him—not the pain, not the fear, not the loss of his faculties or his humanity. I merely sat by and watched. I was the observer of his pain: sitting on the sidelines and wishing I could enter the game, wishing I could run in and be his substitute. I am sick because I felt like I just didn't have the strength or the courage to really put my heart out there enough to try.

I started dating again. It seemed surreal. I always thought I would feel like I was somehow cheating on him, and like it would be weird in an odd way, but it hasn't been. My heart and my mind were too practical to feel that allegiance to someone who was gone.

I found myself going through roller coaster rides of coping. Sometimes I'd drink too much; I'd run too much; I'd cry too much; I'd eat too much, or not enough. It just felt like the only time that I could feel was when it was so intense that I was forced to feel.

I sometimes joked that I have post-traumatic stress disorder, but I don't think that I was really joking. I haven't ever read up on the symptoms, or the reality of what it is all about, but I felt it. I had flashbacks of Colin sitting in his medical bed, a shell of himself—literally skin and bones. In my flashbacks, he's sitting with a computer on his lap: its screen one that I am quite sure he never saw because, in the later days, his vision was well gone. He pretended to look at that computer screen to see a window to the outside world that he was never ready to let go of. He would type away at imaginary pages; pretend to read the news, as he had every day of his life. He would call out to anyone around him and point at things on the screen that were not present. We would all play the game, pretending that we saw what he saw, but anyone who was there was privy to the game. We all knew that whatever reality he was creating was not really there. I'd see him sitting up in his chair, IV pole and medicine behind him pumping away. He would have an eyepatch wrapped around one eye, to reduce the double vision that he was experiencing. But, in all honesty, it never really helped. It was more of a comfort thing, for him to feel like he was doing something. One day, he was sitting with me and messing around with the patch. This was one of the days where he was really despondent, and he was so agitated not to be able to fix his sight or to see something that he so clearly had seen the previous day. He looked at me the way he had begun to—not really at me, but to the side and up: like an old man who had long since lost his sight. He fiddled with his glasses for quite a long time. "Julie!" he shouted at me. "Julie!" as if I was not sitting right next to him. "Julie, I want you to take my glasses into the kitchen and ask Ben to sand them down so that I can see again. I want you to have him sand them down and make them better." I inched closer to him, puzzled as to what he meant, but since these were the days where the hallucinations had become noticeable, I knew instantly that he was talking about something that was not real.

"Colin, I can't do that. There is nothing wrong with your glasses," was my answer to him.

"Julie... I said take my glasses into the kitchen and ask Ben to sand them down so that I can see. You need to do that. You need to fix them so that I can see," he said adamantly.

"Honey, I can't do that... it is not the glasses, sweetheart, it's your eyes. Your eyes are not working properly because you have a tumor that is pressing on your brain," I answered. It had gotten to the point that to sugarcoat anything, to make it sound pleasant or promising or doable, would only bring about further pain for either of us. I had started to see that all of our avoidance of mentioning dying or leaving this earth had begun to feel like I was telling him it was not okay to go. Sitting there, looking at him in those final days, made me only want to beg him to go, to beg him to give up for his own sake, for my sake. I wanted him to accept death, to be okay with it, to be able to pass. My answers to him during this period became very blunt. I felt it would be inhumane not to be. He would sit calmly and nod, appearing to hear and understand what I was saying. "Oh," was usually his answer, with a follow-up about an hour later of "when are we going to go see the eye doctor so I can get new glasses?"

So as I sat there on this particular day with the exact same conversation running—although the addition of the glasses-sanding was new—I just couldn't hold it together. His insistence that I have Ben sand his glasses became more violent, more frustrated, more adamant. "I said go in the kitchen."

"Colin," I finally insistently said forcefully, "you are dying. It is not the glasses. It is the brain tumor that is pressing on your brain. It is getting worse and you are going to die."

"Oh." The agitation disappeared and he shrank back into his chair, placed the eyepatch over the glasses on one eye, and pretended to read the news on the internet again.

Those situations are the ones that I carry with me now. I have so many regrets about the way that I spoke to him, the way that I started to feel as if whatever I said was for naught, as if he was not listening—he was listening, but he was just too scared to acknowledge. Those are the memories which are continually invading my thoughts of our family; the memories of him and I as a couple, as a team, creating this family, living as a family—all of those memories I fight to keep in order to push out the guilt of the illness.

Today was like every other day in our "new" life. The day-to-day has become mundane and uneventful, and I am thankful for that. I have all but forgotten what my life was prior to January of this year. My life is unrecognizable to me. There are so many times that I think everything is okay, that life is okay, and then I catch a glimpse of what life used to be, my life with Colin, and it feels like someone knocked the wind out of me. There is a brief moment of panic—wherein I can't believe that he is no longer here, I can't believe that he is gone—followed by the reality that I am forgetting so quickly what it was like when he was here.

Anyway, as I say, today started out normally. I began listening to the messages on my answering machine. I had decided to go back and to delete the many messages that had built up. I pressed the play button and on came Colin's voice.

"Hi, guys, just wondering where you are . . . I love you."

A wave of emotion rushed over me and before I knew it tears were streaming down my face. I have learned that tears, which I once thought had some voluntary component to them, can happen all on their own without me even realizing.

Matthew looked at me with such worry.

"Matthew, do you know who that was?" I asked him., playing it for him again.

"Uncle Will? Uncle James?" he guessed.

I looked at him and I think I scared him, so I went upstairs to compose myself. I came back minutes later, emotions suppressed, and I said,

"Matthew, that was Daddy."

He had the strangest expression on his face, and then a look of clarity.

"Oh yeah, that was Daddy."

I didn't know whether he actually remembered his voice, but it broke my heart to know that not only am I forgetting him in pieces—but so are they. Coming back to my house this afternoon made me realize *that I have begun to overwrite my old life out of necessity—but that I miss it. I really, really miss it.*

The kids are doing really, really well. I am so proud of how they were able to bond together and lean on each other. Their strength is a true testament to Colin's resilience and love for all of us. Pippa still talks about her daddy often; how he is in heaven and she misses him a lot. Every once in a while, Jake and I can laugh at something he used to do, can remember him, can enjoy the memory without the cloud of sadness that used to wrap itself around everything.

Chapter One—
An Ending And A
New Beginning

I am working on a book that I am writing about Colin and his life, and all of us. Hopefully someday everyone will be able to read of the courage that Colin possessed and the lessons that he taught to everyone he touched. I know it's been a while, but I have not forgotten all that you all have been to us, all that you did for us, all that you continue to do. I just couldn't bring myself to write in this forum again, I couldn't fathom what to say, but the events of the memorial this weekend have catapulted me back in time if for only a brief minute and I just felt compelled to reach out to you all again . . .

I am not sure what lies ahead, but am happy to move forward. Over the past couple of months, I have begun to feel a very fleeting glimpse of hope that my happy ending might be waiting for me somewhere out there. I guess I will just have to wait and see . . . Until next time.

About the Author

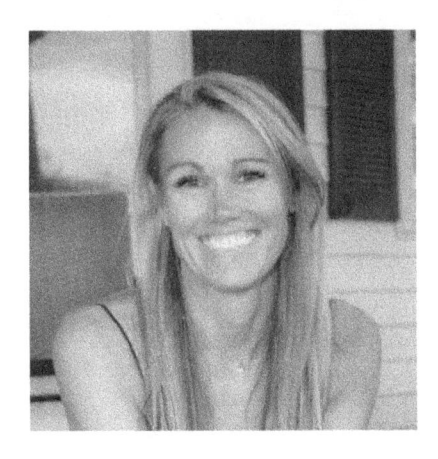

Julie Barth is the mother to six children, who provide her with enough material to sustain her career as a professional writer. Originally from the Midwest, she has been living in South Carolina for over a decade and enjoying the slower-paced life. In her world, truth is truly stranger than fiction. Although some might see her story as tragic and unimaginable, she believes that it is in the hardest moments that the meaning of life reveals itself. Her passion for writing about her own intimate moments and thoughts stems from a desire to help people feel less alone at times when they need support most. There is a saying that "God only gives you what you can handle." Julie believes that sometimes he gives you way more. Sure, "it can always be worse," but what she admits and most won't is "it can sometimes be better." It is okay to be brutally honest, even if it makes others uncomfortable.